DE HISTORIA
UROLOGIAE EUROPAEAE

DE HISTORIA UROLOGIAE EUROPAEAE

VOL. 20

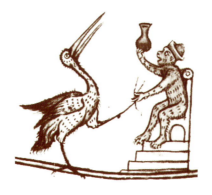

Edited by
Prof. Dr. Dirk Schultheiss

History Office
European Association of Urology
2013

The History Office of the EAU

D. Schultheiss (Chairman)	Giessen (DE)
C. Alamanis	Athens (GR)
J. Elo	Helsinki (FI)
R. Engel (AUA representative)	Linthicum, MD (USA)
L.A. Fariña-Pérez	Vigo (ES)
J.F. Felderhof	The Hague (NL)
A. Figueiredo	Coimbra (PT)
P.P. Figdor	Vienna (AT)
A. Jardin	Paris (FR)
P.E.V. Van Kerrebroeck *(Member-in-waiting)*	Maastricht (NL)
J.J. Mattelaer	Kortrijk (BE)
S. Musitelli (Expert)	Zibidi San Giacomo (IT)
P. Rathert	Düsseldorf (DE)
I. Romics	Budapest (HU)
M. Skopec (Expert)	Vienna (AT)
R. Sosnowski	Warsaw (PL)
P. Thompson	London (GB)
A. Verit	Istanbul (TR)

CONTENTS of VOLUME 20
de Historia Urologiae Europaeae
(2013)

FOREWORD *by Per-Anders Abrahamsson* — 9

INTRODUCTION *by Dirk Schultheiss* — 13

UROLOGICAL THEMES IN ART AND CULTURE

DIEGO RIVERA: HIS ART AND ILLNESS — 15
Jorge Moreno-Palacios, Jorge Moreno-Aranda

CASTRATI: EVERYTHING FOR FAME — 27
Martin Hatzinger

MEDIEVAL UROSCOPY AND URINATING ICONOGRAPHY ON MISERICORDS — 39
Johan J. Mattelaer

FROM "DEVIL'S TEMPTATION" TO "EROTIC IMAGINATION" — 67
Sergio Musitelli, Ilaria Bossi

HISTORICAL TALES IN UROLOGY

DEPICTION OF VENEREAL DISEASES ON WAX MODELS IN THE MOULAGE MUSEUMS OF PARIS AND ATHENS — 81
E. Poulakou-Rebelakou, M. Karamanou, A. Rempelakos, G. Androutsos

PRESIDENT WILSON AND THE MANAGEMENT OF URINARY RETENTION A CENTURY AGO — 91
Jennifer Gordetsky, Ronald Rabinowitz

THE DISCOVERY OF AN EARLY 13TH CENTURY FRAGMENT OF GILLES DE CORBEIL'S CARMINA DE URINARUM IUDICIIS   **101**
Evelien Hauwaerts, Johan R. Boelaert

THE 100TH ANNIVERSARY OF THE JOURNAL D'UROLOGIE MÉDICALE ET CHIRURGICALE   **115**
Johan J. Mattelaer

OPEN CYSTOTOMY FOR BLADDER CANCER   **123**
FROM NECESSITY TO OBSCURITY; THE RISE AND FALL OF A HISTORICAL OPERATION
Susannah M. La-Touche, Roger C. Kockelbergh, Jonathan C. Goddard

UROLOGY IN FRANCE IN THE 19TH CENTURY AND THE BEGINNING OF THE 20TH CENTURY   **137**
AN OVERVIEW OF THE BIRTH OF UROLOGY
Philip E.V. Van Kerrebroeck

RENÉ KÜSS (1913-2006): A TRANSPLANT PIONEER IN PARIS   **181**
Dirk Schultheiss, Alain Jardin

THE AUTHOR RESPONDS: CORRECTIONS TO VOLUME 19   **192**

TABLES OF CONTENTS VOLUMES 1-19   **195**

FOREWORD

An important part of the EAU's identity can be found in the history of our field. Urological conditions have ailed the human race throughout the centuries, and some of the historically most-documented medical conditions are of a urological nature.

In this, the milestone 20th edition of *De Historia Urologiae Europaeae*, we take a look at how urological imagery has permeated culture from the early middle ages to the twentieth century. We learn of the changing artistic interpretation of the *Temptation of St. Anthony* and the increasingly sexual nature of the painters' depiction of said "temptations" over the course of several centuries. It is also interesting to note that images of urination can be found even in the realms of pre-reformation European churches. Mocking uroscopists and representing daily life was a recurrent theme all across Western Europe, as expressed in these architectural flourishes.

This volume also delves into the history of castrati singers, and the medical price they paid for their artistic success. Medical conditions would also manifest themselves in the art of renowned artists. The Mexican painter, mainly known for his expansive murals, Diego Rivera suffered from penile cancer. The subsequent treatment, and the loss of his potency affected him greatly; which he also expressed through his work.

Beside these cultural explorations, this volume also features research into the earliest written descriptions of urological theories and procedures. A remarkable finding in Belgium brought to light a piece of Gilles de Corbeil's, as the parchment it was written on in the 13th century was re-used in a later manuscript. The original fragment gives us a great insight into the state of urological theory in the early middle ages.

The 19th and 20th centuries are approached from a French perspective. Many important steps to establishing urology as a field distinct from surgery were taken in Paris, and we are presented with an exhaustive look of French society, medicine, and finally the development of urology itself. Around this time we also see the foundation of the Journal d'Urologie Médicale et Chirurgicale, which celebrated its centenary last year. *De Historia* includes reproductions of its first pages.

Continuing the importance of France and its urologists for the establishment and development of our field, a tribute to the life and work of transplant pioneer René Küss is also featured. René was a valued colleague, authored several books and was awarded the EAU Willy Gregoir Medal for his achievements in 2002.

More insights into the 19th and 20th centuries come to us from Greece, where a unique collection of urological moulages are on display. The state of treatment of urinary retention at the beginning of the 20th century is examined through the fascinating story of President Woodrow Wilson's medical history. We also look at the history of open cystotomy, and its changing prominence as a technique for treating bowel cancer.

I would like to thank the EAU History Office for another worthy addition to a long-running series. Each year brings new insights, new contributors and new areas of research. I hope you enjoy reading it!

PER-ANDERS ABRAHAMSSON
EAU Secretary General

INTRODUCTION

Welcome to the 20th Volume of *De Historia Urologiae Europaeae*! This certainly represents a milestone for the EAU and its History Office, and I am pleased to preside over this anniversary. This volume contains a wide range of articles, with a particular interest for urological themes in art and culture. There is also a clear French theme. This is the result of last year's Annual EAU Congress taking place in Paris.

After editing the very first volume of *De Historia* in 1994, at 20 volumes it is time for the EAU History Office to bid farewell to Johan Mattelaer. We thank him for all of his efforts over the years, and hope to continue receiving his contributions for our publications. One of his publications, *Sexological and other Less Logical Stories* is a gift for EAU members at the 28th Annual EAU Congress in Milan.

Johan's seat in the office will be filled by his countryman Phillip Van Kerrebroeck at the next History Office Meeting, to be held in the autumn of 2013. Appropriately, it will be held in Belgium. Both have featured articles in this volume of *De Historia*.

We had a wealth of excellent articles to choose from this year, so regrettably we were not able to include all of them. Your submissions are first in line for consideration for inclusion in Volume 21. Thank you, as always, to the reviewers and experts of the EAU History Office who offered their expertise during the editing process.

Dirk Schultheiss
EAU History Office Chairman

DIEGO RIVERA: HIS ART AND ILLNESS

Jorge Moreno-Palacios[1], Jorge Moreno-Aranda[2]

1. Hospital de Especialidades CMN S XXI, Department of Urology, Mexico City, Mexico.

2. Hospital Angeles del Pedregal, Chairman of Surgery Department, Mexico City, Mexico.

1

March, G. and D. Rivera. My Art, My Life: An Autobiography. Citadel Press: New York, 1960.

The Beginning

Diego Rivera Barrientos was born on December 13, 1886 in Guanajuato, México. Already at an early age, he showed an ability for drawing; his father's friends nicknamed him "The Engineer".[1] At the age of thirteen, Rivera was accepted at the San Carlos Academy of Art (as the youngest student in its history) in Mexico City. Its director was the classic painter Santiago Rebull (1829-1902). Diego's good work won him a scholarship from the Mexican Government to study in Spain from 1907 to 1910 in the studio of the Spanish painter, Eduardo Chicharro.

During his first journey to Europe, Rivera was influenced greatly by impressionist and postimpressionist painters. After a short trip to Mexico to present his first art exposition, he returned to Paris and lived in Montparnasse. He became a figure in the Cubism movement, and mixed with numerous artists, like Amadeo Modigliani, Marevna Vorobieff, Chaïm Soutine, Pablo Picasso and Max Jacob, among others.

He married for the first time, to the Russian painter Angelina Beloff, and had a son named Diego Maria. His son would die of meningitis in the first year of his life. Rivera was nearly 30 at the time, and by then he had arrived to the masterly zenith of his Cubist phase. He was invited by the Mexican Government to execute a series of frescoes in the country. These frescoes were to be part of an educational program to show, through his paintings, the history of Mexico to its people.

Rivera spent the last months of his stay in Europe, in Italy, where he learnt the techniques of mural painting through the works of Giotto and Michelangelo.[2]

[2] Tirado, J.R. and L. García. *Genios del Arte*, Diego Rivera. Susaeta: Barcelona, 2004.

Mexico, Rivera's Eternal Love
In 1922, Rivera painted his first fresco in the Amphitheatre Simón Bolivar, at the National Preparatory School, the upper school of former College of San Ildelfonso in Mexico City. Here, he would meet Frida Kahlo, a young student. The name of the mural was "The Creation", and one of the models for this mural was Guadalupe Marin, who became his second wife and the mother of his two daugthers, Guadalupe and Ruth. This is a work in which Nazarene stylistic elements are evident, and in the execution of which Rivera found his Italian studies of a great use.[3]

[3] Kettenmann, A. *Rivera*. Taschen: Köln, 2006.

Rivera was also known for his communist ideas, which he expressed in numerous frescoes. Together with the Mexican painter David Alfaro Siqueiros, he published the leftist newspaper *The Machete*, which was the official organ of the Mexican Communist Party.

From 1923 to 1928, he painted around 5,000 square meters in 124 frescoes in the building of The Ministry of Public Education, in Mexico City. This was the largest project of the mural movement in Mexico. The thematic programme for the murals consists of motifs of revolutionary ideals, descriptions of the everyday life for Mexican people (scenes of rural, industrial and art craft activities) and scenes of traditional Mexican folk parties.

Sexuality was a very important part of Diego Rivera's life. A variety of sexual motifs are shown in his work. This expression is clear in the frescoes painted for The National Agricultural School in Chapingo, Mexico. One example comes from the cycle "Song to Earth (Natural Evolution)" which includes the frescoes Germination, Maturation, Fecundation and Underground Forces. In these frescoes, Diego shows numerous nude figures of women with great sensuality (and subliminal phallic forms). One of the models for this mural was the Italian-American photographer Tina Modotti.[4] (Figs. 1 and 2)

4

Lozano LM, J.R. Coronel-Rivera. *Diego Rivera: Obra Mural Completa*. Taschen: Köln 2008.

Figure 1: Fecundation, 1926, fresco, Universidad Autónoma de Chapingo, Texcoco, México

Figure 2: The Phallus, detail on a window, from the fresco Fecundation, 1926, Universidad Autónoma de Chapingo, Texcoco, México.

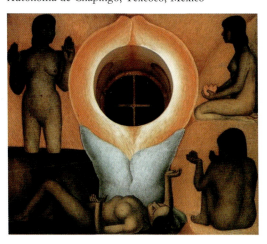
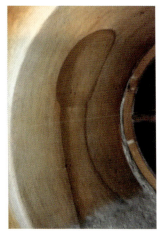

From Mexico to the World

In 1929, Rivera married the young Mexican painter Frida Kahlo. They were a singular couple known for their liberal ideas about love. Also in 1929, Rivera was invited to the United States for the first time to paint a mural at the California School of Fine Arts. After that, he was obliged to return to México to finish his work at Mexico City's National Palace.

Soon after his return, he was invited to perform a large scale exhibition at the Museum of Modern Art in New York, as only the second painter after Henri Matisse to have a one-man exhibition. After he finished his exhibition in New York, he was invited by Edsel B. Ford (son of Henry Ford) to paint the interior walls of The Detroit Institute of Arts (from 1932 to 1933). According to Rivera, this is one of his masterpieces and the most strenuous job that he had ever done.[2]

As one of the most famous artists in the United States, Rivera was invited by the Rockefeller family along with Picasso and Matisse to paint a fresco at The Rockefeller Center. Only Rivera accepted the invitation. As part of the fresco "Man at the Crossroads, looking with Hope and High Vision to the Choosing of a New and Better Future", he painted a portrait of Vladimir Lenin. This painting proved controversial in the conservative community. Nelson and John Rockefeller, the clients' representatives, negotiated with Rivera to remove the portrait, but he refused. The artist was paid off and released from his obligation, and the mural was subsequently destroyed.

Rivera, now in Mexico painted an almost identical version of the New York mural at the Palace of Fine Arts in Mexico City, named "Man, Controller of the Universe". As an expression of his disapproval, Diego painted Nelson Rockefeller beside the bacteria that represent the venereal diseases in the mural.[2]

In 1937, Mexico gave asylum to Leon Trotsky and his wife. They were received at the Kahlo's House (at the time, Frida and Diego were divorced after he had had an affair with Frida's sister) where they stayed for the next two years. During that time, Diego and Frida also received André Breton, one of the leaders of the surrealist movement. He was an important influence in the international projection of Frida Kahlo's work worldwide. After escalating differences of opinion with Rivera, Trotsky moved out from Kahlo's house, and he was murdered on Joseph Stalin's orders in August, 1940, by the Spanish communist and Soviet agent Ramon Mercader.[5]

Diego was a friend of the Mexican cardiologist Ignacio Chavez, who asked Rivera in 1943 to paint two murals for the National Institute of Cardiology. For this work, Rivera, conducted thorough research on the history of cardiology through the ages. His murals spanned a total area of 48.9 m^2, and featured all of the scientists who had made contributions to the development of cardiology (Galen, Malpighi, Harvey, Auenbrugger, Laennec, Aschoff, His, Röntgen, Einthoven amongst others). Rivera remarried Kahlo in December, 1940. They decided to live in separate houses, share expenses and ideas, but with no physical contact.[6]

5
Valle P. *Grandes Pintores, Diego Rivera*. Editorial Epoca: Mexico City, 2006.

6
Billeter, E. *Das Blaue Haus: Die Welt der Frida Kahlo*. Schrin Kunsthalle: Germany, 1993.

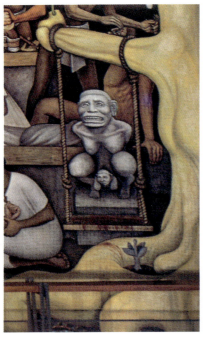

Figure 3: Green Tree of Life, detail of the fresco The People's Demand for a Better Health,1953, Fresco, Hospital de la Raza, Mexico City, Mexico.

Figure 4: Evening Twightlight No 8, 1956, oil and tempera on canvas, Dolores Olmedo Museum, Mexico City, Mexico.

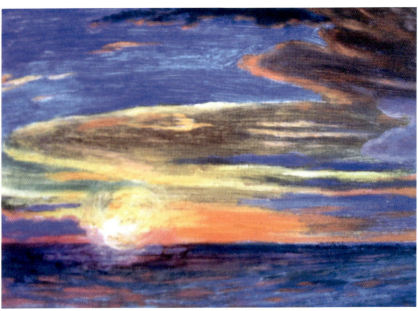

His Illness

In 1952, Rivera was bothered by a pain in the penis and he had urinary retention, the diagnosis was penile cancer. His doctors at that time were Ignacio Millán (an oncologist) and Manuel Aceves (a pathologist). As a first treatment, a penectomy with orchiectomy was offered but he refused. He told the doctor, "I want everything to remain as it is. I will be completely responsible. I refuse to allow the amputation of those organs which have given me the finest pleasure I know." Diego Rivera underwent X-Ray treatments in Mexico from May to June 1952, with apparent good results.[2]

The fresco "The People's Demand for a Better Health" in the *Hospital de la Raza*, Mexico City, shows the expression of his suffering; in it he exhibits a giant phallic, yellow-green Tree of Life. After finishing it he thought "No more for me. Physical love exists for me no longer. I am an old man, too old, too sick, to enjoy that wonderful ecstasy."[2] The mural's central image shows the aztec godess *Tlazeotl* (deity of life and labour), and Rivera makes a tribute to pre-Hispanic native medicine, as well as medical advances, represented by Pierre and Marie Curie. (Fig. 3)

After a long period of illness, Frida Kahlo died in July 1954, and with her, so did Diego's partner, art critic, companion, lover and friend.

Treatment in Russia

In 1955, Diego married Emma Hurtado, a personal friend and owner of an art gallery. They were invited to the International Peace Congress in Europe. On that journey, Diego visited Poland, Czechoslovakia, and Russia.[7] He

---
7
Rivera Marin, G. *Encuentros con Diego Rivera*. México, 2004.

was admitted to the fifth pavilion of the S.P. Botkin hospital in Moscow, from September 12, 1955 to January 21, 1956. Professor A.P. Frumkin was in charge of his case. Upon his admission, the doctors described a vegetant and ulcerated lesion in the inner face of the prepuce with important oedema and an ulcer of 0.8 by 0.8 cm beside the frenulum, at that time no inguinal lymph nodes were involved.

Russian doctors proposed as a treatment: brachytherapy, external beam radiation and adjuvant surgery. Rivera, underwent brachytherapy from September 22 to 27, with a total dose of 5,100 cGy in 4 fractions. Subsequently, he had external beam radiotherapy for one week, receiving 3,000 cGy. After certain regression of the lesion, Professor A.P. Frumkin and colleagues decided with Rivera's approval to perform a circumcision. The surgery was performed on October 20, using ether and oxygen as anesthetics, surgical margin was the tunica albuginea and catgut was used as suture. The hystopathological analysis showed a grainy ulcer with sclerosis, on the microscope picnotic and atypical cells suspicious of epidermoid carcinoma were found.[8]

Rivera remained in hospital under medical surveillance until January, 1956, making numerous drawings during his hospital stay.

Diego's Sunset

Upon his return from Russia, Diego was received by Dolores Olmedo Patiño, with whom he spent some days at her home, known as *El Batan* in Mexico City. During his stay, Diego continued his treatment in Mexico, with Oncologist Dr. Guillermo Montaño. He

8
Unpublished. Diega Rivera's Medical History, located at the Dolores Olmedo Museum.

presented a recurrence of his cancer on the right groin, where inguinal lymph nodes were involved; receiving external beam radiotherapy with a dose of 4,000 cGy in 20 fractions.[9]

During his stay with Dolores Olmedo, Rivera was invited to spend a short time in Acapulco, Mexico, painting numerous sunsets in oil, in which, despite being in the decline of his life, he demonstrated his extraordinary artistic quality and genius. (Fig. 4)

On September, 1957, Diego suffered a cerebrovascular disease, which left in him as a sequel, paralysis of his right arm and impeding him to continue painting. This sent him into a state of severe depression.[7] He asked to be moved to his art studio, surrounded by pre-Hispanic icons and idols (of which he was a great collector) and two easels with unfinished paintings. One of them depicted his granddaughter and the other a smiling Russian girl. He spent his final days in his studio.[10]

He died of a heart failure in his studio on November 24, 1957. Rivera wanted to be cremated and his ashes put together with those of Frida Kahlo. Against his will, by orders of the Mexican President, Adolfo Ruiz Cortines, he was buried at the "Rotunda of Illustrious Men" in recognition of his extraordinary artistic work.

Conclusions

Diego Rivera is perhaps the most important painter of the Mexican mural movement. Through his frescoes in Mexico, San Francisco, Detroit and the Rockefeller Center in New York, he reached worldwide fame.

---

9 Personal interview with Dr. Casab, Radiotherapy Fellow of Dr. Guillermo Montaño.

10 Wolfe, BD. *La Fabulosa Vida de Diego Rivera*. México, 1972. 329-330.

Sexuality was a very important part of his life, integrating diverse kinds of sexual motifs and imagery in his work. He was diagnosed with penile cancer, treated according to the knowledge of the disease at that time, and he expressed his illness in his art.

D.R. © 2012 Banco de México, "Fiduiciario" en el Fideicomiso relativo a los Museos Diego Rivera y Frihda Khalo. Av. 5 de Mayo No 2., Col Centro, Del. Cuahutémoc 06059, México, D.F and Reproducción autorizada por el Instituto Nacional de Bellas Artes y literatura, 2012.

Correspondence to:
Jorge Moreno Palacios
Department of Urology
Hospital de Especialidades CMN Siglo XXI.
Av. Cuauhtémoc 330, Col. Doctores, CP 06720
Del. Cuauhtémoc, México City.
E-Mail: jorgemorenomd@gmail.com

CASTRATI: EVERYTHING FOR FAME

Martin Hatzinger[1]

1. Chief of the minimal invasive department Markushospital Frankfurt/Main, Germany

In the middle of the sixteenth century, castration in connection with singing became widespread in Europe, especially in Italy. Eight- to nine-year-old boys were castrated before they reached puberty so that their voices did not break. This procedure was practised by so-called 'Norcinis', who were virtually only unskilled village quacks specialising in castration. Castration was performed without disinfection and under primitive conditions with a special set of instruments appropriately called 'Castratori'. Many a child died a painful death from wound infection or profuse loss of blood.

The procedure was performed in strict secrecy as it was forbidden under canon law with the threat of excommunication for those concerned. Those boys who outlived the procedure were given a stringent musical education that generally lasted around eight years. This meant that firstly, their musical debut did not take place until they were in their twenties and secondly they commanded a singing technique that would still fill today's modern singers with envy.

The physical effects

The effects of castration on physical development were notoriously erratic, as the Ottoman eunuchs in the Seraglio of Constantinople knew. Much depended on the timing of the operation: boys pruned before the age of ten or so very often grew up with feminine features, smooth, hairless bodies, incipient breasts, infantile penis and often a complete lack of sex drive. But those castrated after the age of ten, as puberty encroached, could continue to develop physically and often sustain sufficient erections.

Often castration is associated with a marked decrease in libido and erectile function [1,2]. However we know from modern studies that 25% of castrated patients after orchiectomy respond to visual erotic stimulation with functional erection.[3] The human adrenal gland is a source of peripherally circulating androgen precursors, thus complete androgen insufficiency may not be observed in men at a younger age.[4]

Gender confusion

The castrati were designated to take female roles in opera as during the baroque era, as it was not becoming for women to take part themselves. The 'Primo uomo' was the equivalent of today's primadonna. He and the 'Secundo uomo', usually also a castrato, were the chief singers in almost all 'Opera seria'.[5] The imitation of the female sex was physically emphasised by the obvious testosterone deficiency that led to breast growth and a similar fat distribution to that in females, thus causing great irritation and controversy all around. For example, in his memoirs, Casanova wrote: "In order not to succumb to temptation it is wise to keep as cool and sensible as a German".[6]

One of the most confusing moments in Casanova's life came when he met a lovely teenage castrato named Bellino. Casanova was bewitched, going so far as to offer a gold doubloon to see the boy's genitals. In an improbable twist, when Casanova grabbed Bellino in a fit

1
Brett, M.A., L.F. Roberts, T.W. Jonhson, R.J. Wassersurg. "Eunuchs in contemporary society : Expectations, consequences and adjustments to castration." *J Sex Med.* 2007; 4 : 946-955.

2
Roberts, L.F., M.A. Brett, T.W. Johnson, R.J. Wassersurg. "Passion for castration: Characterizing men who are fascinated with castration, but have not been castrated." *J Sex Med.* 2008; 5: 1669-1680.

3
Greenstein, A, S.R. Plymate and P.G. Katz. "Visually stimulated erection in castrated men." *J Urol.* 153, 650-652.

4
Traish, A.M. and A.T. Guay. "Are androgens critical for penile erections in humans? Examining the clinical and preclinical evidence." *J Sex Med.* 2006;3:382-407.

5
Haböck, F. *Die Kastraten und ihre Gesangskunst. Eine gesangsphysiologische, kultur- und musikhistorische Studie.* Deutsche Verlagsanstalt: Stuttgart, Berlin and Leipzig, 1927.

6
Casanova, G. *Memoires - Histoire de ma vie, vol. 10.* Brussels, 1838.

of passion, he discovered a false penis: it turned out that the castrato was a girl. She had taken up to disguise to circumvent the ban on female singers in Italy. The pair became lovers, but Casanova dumped her later in Venice.

In the seventeenth and eighteenth century, it was possible for castrated males to gain international fame and become superstars. The young singers, mainly from the lower classes, not only associated with popes, emperors, kings and aristocracy, but also with prostitutes and common folk. They did not all manage to handle their fame and glory adroitly and embarassing incidents and total decline were not seldom. They had started singing at an early age and their career was sometimes only short, ending at the latest around the age of fifty. Caffarelli bought himself a duchy, Senesino fought a running battle with his family, Bernacchi founded a singing school, and the most famous of them all, Farinelli, retired to Bologna and learned to play the viola da gamba.

All this can be put down to the fault of the church. Paul's letter to the Corinthians was interpreted to convey the meaning that women had no say in church affairs: "Mulier taceat in ecclesia". What actually was meant was that women were unsuitable as preachers. The ecclesiasts themselves decided that women were to be additionally excluded from any kind of music. As a result, only men were allowed to sing in the choirs of the papal chapel. Boys or male falsetto voices sang the high-scale roles.[7]

Singing technique

It was suddenly discovered that the boys' voices did not break at all after castration.

---

[7] Deuster, C. "How did the castratos sing? Historical observations." *Wurzbg Medizinhist Mitt.* 2006; 25: 133-152.

Although strictly forbidden by canon law, they were quite willing to bear all risks for the sake of fame and glory. Only few possessed voices that satisfied the high demands of the audience. But those talented ones with angelic voices filled the audience with rapture. Today, we can only vaguely speculate on how these androgynous figures really felt, both physically and emotionally. We know from contemporary studies that the major sexual effects are the loss of libido, hot flashes and genital shrinkag.[1, 2]

The majority of castrati did not experience a successful singing career and their mutilation caused havoc in the attempt to lead a normal life. Castration not only affected their vocal cords, but also their whole further physical development. Important hormones were missing at a vital stage of physical development. Many became extremely tall and fat – they were more or less giants with a childlike voice.[8, 9]

The most important duty of the singing teachers was to meltingly combine a sonorous chest-voice with a softer sounding falsetto. The sublime castrato voice was a synthesis of these two types of voices. A larynx the size of a child combined with the lung volume of an adult male produced a strong, radiating chest-voice excelling that of a natural female or male voice. A really sonorous depth is therefore missing in normal males with falsetto voices (countertenors).

Descriptions given by numerous contempories of that time give us only a slight idea of how the castrati' voices really sounded. Some authors report on a male timbre, others compare them to a deep female voice. No matter

8
Jenkins, J.S. "The lost voice: A history of the castrato", *J. Pediatr Endocrinol Metab.* 2000; 13 Suppl 6: 1503-1508.

9
Melicow, M.M. and S. Pulrang. "Castrati choir and opera singers". *Urology* 1974; May; 3 (5): 663-670.

what, their most unusual physical appearance, their extraordinary voices coupled with the extremely difficult voice acrobatics demanded by the baroque opera that entailed endless warbling, improvisation and long-held tones, electrified and fascinated the audience.[7]

Castrati in society

Society in the eighteenth century considered castrati to be a disturbing ambiguous and contradictory phenomenon. The fact that castrati could enjoy sexual relationship without the obvious consequences caused less sarcasm than worry amongst the contemporary men. The sterility of the castrati was not considered a disqualification from society, but a definite triumph. Most castrati never even attempted to contradict the rumours on their legendary virility.

In our days there are although a large group of men who are fascinated with castration, but have not been castrated. Many only fantasize; others realize their fantasies. Motivating factors are the feeling of calmness, the control of sexual urges and appetite, the sexual thrill of a sadomasochistic nature and a castration paraphilia.[1, 2]

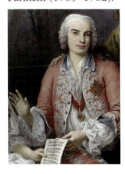

Figure 1:
Carlo Broschi, alias Farinelli (1705–1782).

Farinelli

Carlo Broschi, alias Farinelli (1705–1782; Fig. 1), was undoubtedly the most famous singer of his time. Technically incomparable, he nevertheless remained extremely modest and his incredible popularity would make many a popstar today envious. Musically, he was educated by the famous Maestro Porpora in Naples. He celebrated his debut in 1720 at the age of fifteen. He performed at almost all principalities

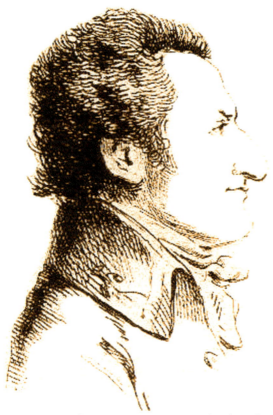

Figure 2:
Gaetano Majorano,
alias Caffareli.

in Europe with great success. At the height of fame, he sang in London at the opera of the nobility to full houses and with unbounded triumph. Farinelli left London in 1737 when he was called to Spain by Queen Elisabetta Farnese in the hope that his singing would heal the depression suffered by her husband, King Philipp V.

This early example of musical therapy turned out to be so effective that Farinelli stayed for 22 years at the Spanish court. He was on very close terms with the king and soon became the most influential man in Spain. In due course he founded an Italian opera society there and was given the position of a minister. Each evening, he sang the same four opera arias exclusively for King Philipp.

Under the reign of Philipp's successor, King Ferdinand VI, he still held the same position and title and it was not until the reign of the next king, Charles III that he was dismissed in 1759 following a scheming campaign instigated by Charles' mother. Up to his departure he had amassed a considerable fortune with which he retired to Bologna in 1760, where he was visited by such people as Charles Burney, Casanova and the young Mozart. After his death in 1782, he was buried in accordance with his wishes on a hill near Bologna following a simple ceremony.[5, 10, 11, 12]

10
Barbier, P. *Farinelli: Le castrat des Lumieres*. Grasset: Paris, 1994.

11
Jenkins, J.S. "The voice of the castrato." *Lancet*. 1998, Jun 20; 351 (9119): 1877-1880.

12
Ortkemper, H. *Engel wider Willen. Die Welt der Kastraten; eine andere Operngeschichte*. Hentschel Verlag: Berlin, 1993.

Caffarelli

Caffarelli was born under the name of Gaetano Majorano in 1710 in Bitonto near Bari (Fig. 2). At the age of nine, his father took him to the town of Norcia in Umbria to have him castrated. As they were unknown in this town it was easy to keep the castration a secret. During the seventeenth and eighteenth century, the lonely town in the hills was known to be one of the centres for castration in Italy. All the medics and quacks who performed castration were therefore referred to as 'Norcini'.

Caffarelli was also musically educated in Naples by Master Porpora, who finally said to him: "I dismiss you now, my son, as I have taught you all I know. You are now the greatest singer in Italy and the whole world". He was indeed triumphantly celebrated throughout Europe, but he always stood in close competition to Farinelli. It was not until Farinelli went to the Spanish court that Caffarelli gained fame in his own rights. Just the same as all preceding castrati and those who came after him, he celebrated his greatest success in London. He performed brilliantly in several operas composed by Händel at the Haymarket Theatre and enraptured the audience with his voice.

Despite his fame, he was also notorious for his violent temper and outrageous arrogance. For example, he disdainfully rejected a snuffbox presented to him by Louis XV after one of his performances in Paris as being unworthy. The very next day Caffarelli was exiled from France. He fought once with one of his colleagues in a church during a performance and was consequently charged for blasphemy and sent to prison.

Finally, in 1755 he settled in Naples and purchased a duchy there, a clear indication that the existence as a castrato could be very lucrative. He had the following inscription mounted on his town mansion: "Amphion Thebas, ego Domum" (Amphion built Thebes, I built this house). This was later wittily supplemented by the words "Ille cum, tu sine" (He with, you without). During his last years he often performed for charity and also supported the poor. He died in 1783 in Naples and was buried in the San Efremo monaster.[12, 13]

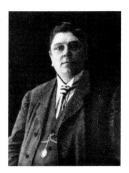

Figure 3: Alessandro Moreschi.

13

Koldau, L. "Ille cum, tu sine. Der Kampf um die Männlichkeit bei den Kastraten des 18. Jahrhunderts." 2nd. meeting AIM Gender; 7-9 Nov. 2002. Stuttgart, Germany.

Alessandro Moreschi

Alessandro Moreschi (Fig. 3) was one of the last castrati and the only one from whom recordings of his voice still exist today. He commenced with singing lessons at the age of thirteen at the Scuola di San Salvatore. After completing his musical education he joined the choir of the Sistine Chapel and advanced to soloist and finally choir leader. Following the ban on castration enforced by Pope Pius X, all castrati were eventually dismissed and replacements found. Moreschi retired in 1912 after thirty years choir membership.

Those recordings made by Moreschi from 1902 to 1904 that still exist today only allow us to perceive the extraordinary virtuosity and extensive scope of the castrati voices during the eighteenth century. These recordings transmit the sound of a castrato, which is clearly quite different to that of modern counter-tenors. Moreschi was given the nickname 'Angelo di Roma'.

In 1914, Prof. Franz Haböck, a well-known German researcher on castrati, had planned with Moreschi to stage a hommage to Farinelli, the most famous of all castrati. Unfortunately it turned out that Moreschi's voice was not good enough to realise this project. The reason for this was probably the fact that his musical education was based on the ideals of the nineteenth century. It was not possible for him to master the difficult parts sung by Farinelli. [5, 7, 9, 14]

14
Clapton, N. *Moreschi: The Angel of Rome, The voice of the castrato*. Haus Publishing Limited: London, 2008.

Händel

When talking about the phenomena of castrated singers, one must surely talk of Georg Friedrich Händel (1685-1759). His artistic work as composer of innumerable operas and oratories, and as director of the Covent Garden theatre and Queen's theatre, very closely connected him with the destiny of the castrati of those times (Fig. 4). The bankruptcy of his theatres as well as his death in 1759 started the slow downfall of the former superstars.

The last production of an opera composed by Georg Friedrich Händel (1685–1759) was in 1755 in London. With the exception of the "Messiah", his operas gradually disappeared from the stages of the world. The same applied to the once fashionable castrati; female singers took over their roles whilst the tenors became the new heroes of opera. The last known opera in which a castrato played was Mayerbeers "Il Crociato in Egitto" in 1824. The last official performance by a castrato in London was dated to be 1844.

Conclusion

On stage, the castrati were celebrated stars, in the salons of the nobility they were welcomed as prominent personalities, but as individuals they were despised and discriminated. Marriage with a castrato was scorned and forbidden as they were infertile, but two singers in Germany did acquire special legal dispensation to remain in wedlock. In one of these cases the famous castrato Bartolomeo de Sorlisi gained 1666 in Dresden the permission to marry his fiancée, but after three different expertises and a long dishonourable law process the love affair ended tragically with the early death of the husband.[9] It was common for women to flatter them and flirt with them and to even take them as lovers, but marriage with a castrato was strictly forbidden – moral hypocrisy in a gallant era.

Adult men with angelic voices would sound strange to us nowadays, but in the baroque era, they were acclaimed superstars.

Nowadays, only the polished singing technique counts and not the surgeon's knife. Out of one hundred castrated boys, only one conserved his beautiful young voice and again, only a minority of these actually became famous international singers. During the baroque era, when the audience frenetically celebrated the performance of the 'Primo uomo' they did not shout "Bravo" or "Bravissimo", but "Eviva il cotello": *long live the knife*.

Correspondence to:
Dr. Martin Hatzinger
Department of Urology
Chief of the minimal invasive department
Markushospital Frankfurt/Main, Germany
Wilhelm-Epstein-Strasse 4
60431 Frankfurt
E-Mail: martin.hatzinger@fdk.info

MEDIEVAL UROSCOPY AND URINATING ICONOGRAPHY ON MISERICORDS

Johan J. Mattelaer[1]

1. *Urologist in Kortrijk, Belgium, Member of the History Office of the EAU*

Misericords

Carved misericords are one of the most fascinating, yet perhaps least understood aspects of medieval art. The word *misericord* comes from the Latin word for mercy and sums up the purpose of these wooden seats succinctly. The offices of the medieval church were rigorous with 8 services held daily: Matins, Lauds, Prime, Terce, Sext, Nones, Vespers and Compline, each with the recitation of psalms, canticles and hymns. Such rituals were physically demanding as the participants stood for most of the time, often with their arms raised.

From the end of the 12th century onwards, seats were introduced into the choir stalls which, when raised for standing, provided a small projecting upper ledge upon which the occupant could rest while remaining upright through the long hours of prayer. The consoles of these load-bearing blocks of wood provided ideal surfaces for carving.

From the 13th century many of the consoles were decorated with recognisable religious subjects but a large number also showed mythical beasts and scenes from the comic to the profane and even the obscene. These include stories of animals mimicking human behaviour, assorted fables (often about Reynard the Fox), incidents of domestic strife (women thrashing men), proverbs, scenes of daily life and faces known as images of the 'green man'.[1]

From 1250 until 1550, before the Reformation, misericords were found throughout Western Europe, with the exception of Italy. We studied these misericord carvings and found a large number that represent uroscopy and scenes of urination. This paper is an overview of our findings. Almost all of the satirical carvings of uroscopy with ape-doctors are to be found in England, while normal scenes of a physician-uroscopist and urinating scenes are more usual in continental Europe.

Not all misericords are to be found in monastic churches: they are also present in parish churches, secular cathedrals and university college chapels. A large number of the misericords feature obscene images. Many writers have explained these as 'moralising' images of deadly sins (although this sometimes stretches belief). Another argument is that the purpose was to sanctify the everyday -even the profane- by bringing it right into the choir of the church.

We still tend to see the Middle Ages through the filter of Victorian Christianity, but in fact, there were not the same taboos. Monks may have taken vows of chastity, but there were clearly many who had taken such religious vows -including plenty of clergy, too- who did not see a contradiction between the patronage of these images and their spirituality.

It has sometimes been argued that these 'profane' images are on misericords precisely because of their position -beneath the bottoms of the worshipers- but this argument does not

[1] Hardwick Paul, *English Medieval Misericords: The Margins of Meaning*, The Boydell Press, 2011.

seem to hold water: misericords are also known to feature images of the resurrected Christ, and the Coronation of the Virgin.

Medieval churches were not just places of worship: they stood at the heart of many medieval communities, and perhaps it was thought fitting that their iconography should reflect all of the community's activities. Of course, humour also played an important role.

There was already a debate on this matter at the time. Bernard of Clairvaux had already chastised the church patrons for the "comely deformity" of the grotesques on the outside of churches, well before the first misericords were carved in England in the thirteenth century. But it seems that his voice was in the minority.

There is also the 'pagan counterculture' argument. Iconographically, some of these images (the shee-la-na-gig and the green man being the two most obvious examples) clearly have pagan origins. Medieval Catholicism was a syncretistic religion, in the sense that when it came to Western Europe, it absorbed existing pagan elements rather than obliterating them. This legacy was, of course, what the Puritans would object to in the later history of the Church, and that is why many of these images have been damaged.

Another element that also inspires some of these images is satire based on very localised needs. Thus, in a monastic church, the fox to geese will almost certainly be in the garb of a preaching friar, and not of a monk. (Fig. 1) The satire on doctors, as we will see below, is another example.

Dozens of books have sought to explain these scenes. Suggestions include the church giving free rein to carvers to show their skills, the desire to amuse monks on cold nights, or even early instances of toilet humour, since people literally sat with their bottoms on the carvings.

Uroscopy

The primary iconographic symbol of the physician in the later medieval period (1300-1500 AD) is the distinctive uroscopy flask: the *matula* or *jordan*. It was the most important diagnostic tool employed by the medieval medical doctor. Colour, quality, smell and sedimentary deposits of the patients' urine were analysed, often with the help of elaborate reference charts [2].

We can see a doctor portrayed as a uroscopist on misericords in Breda and Bruges. (Figs. 2 and 3) Uroscopy is also depicted on a misericord in the Great Malvern Priory, St Mary and St Michael's, Worcestershire, where a sick man is supported by a woman while a doctor looks at two urine flasks, which he holds in his hands. (Fig. 4) It can likewise be found on the woodcarvings in St Mary's, Bury St Edmunds, Suffolk. In Spain, uroscopy is shown on a panel in the choir stalls of the cathedral at Sevilla (Fig. 5) and in Léon Cathedral.

The art of uroscopy involved the visual inspection of urine in a specially shaped flask called a matula. By the 14th century it had become an integral part of the assessment of the patient's humoral balance, which was the linchpin of both diagnosis and management in medieval medical practice. The matula became the symbol of a physician: *Matula fecit medicus*.

[2] Mattelaer, J.J. *Uroscopy in: Europe, The Cradle of Urology.* Chapter 3.1., EAU History Office: Arnhem, 2010.

So ingrained is the iconography of the urine flask that it even occurs in the famous illustration of Chaucer's Physician in the Ellesmere manuscript of the *Canterbury Tales*: (Fig. 6)

> *I pray to God so save thy gentil cors,*
> *and eek thyne urynals and thy jurdones,*
> *thyn ypocras, and eek thy galiones,*
> *and every boyste ful of letuarie*[3]

However, the practice was open to abuse by unscrupulous physicians, who offered treatment solely on the basis of uroscopy, without even seeing the patient. Further abuse occurred when Latin texts on the subject were translated into the vernacular by unqualified imposters. Although more orthodox practitioners and physicians tried hard to distance themselves from such practices, by the 15th century the art of uroscopy was falling into disrepute and the matula became a symbol of ridicule.[4]

On the carved misericordes in choir stalls, the physician holding the matula was commonly represented as an ape, with the allegorical implications of foolishness, vanity and even lechery. The ape uroscopist was frequently shown with his friend the fox, an animal that was often used to satirise the less-than-perfect cleric. This association may reflect the close ties between the medical and clerical professions in the late medieval period. As David A. Sprunger notes: *with their physical resemblance to humans and their capacity to mimic but not understand behaviour, apes have long been used for human parody.*[5]

Satire took a back seat to sermonising. Medieval preachers often likened Christ and the Church to, who cured men's souls.[5] The

---

[3] Chaucer G., *The Canterbury Tales*, in *The Riverside Chaucer*, VI 304-307, ed. L.D. Benson, Oxford, 1988.

[4] Connor H. "Medieval uroscopy and its representation on misericords, part 1: Uroscopy." *Clin. Med.* 1 (6), p.507-9, 2001 and part 2: 2 (1), 75-7, 2002.

[5] Sprunger, D.A. "Parodic animal physicians from the margins of medieval manuscripts," in: *Animals in the Middle Ages*, 67-81, ed. N.C. Flores. London, 1996.

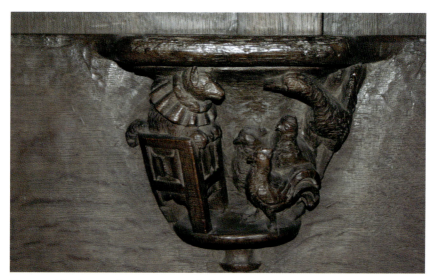

Figure 1: The fox preaching to geese will almost certainly be in the garb of a preaching friar, and not of a monk. Misericord in Manchester Cathedral. © Johan J. Mattelaer

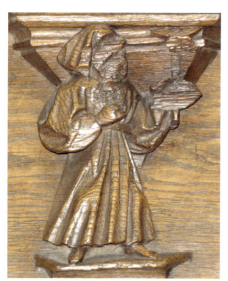

Figure 2: Doctor examining urine (damaged). Misericord in the 'Grote Kerk' (Church of Our Lady), Breda, The Netherlands
© Johan J. Mattelaer

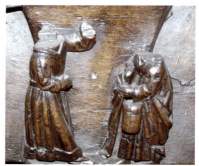

Figure 3: Doctor examining urine. The matula in his left hand is missing, but we can clearly see the specific bag in woven straw used to protect the fragile matula when bringing the urine for uroscopy (hanging on the left arm of the woman). Misericord in St. Salvator Church, Bruges.
© Johan J. Mattelaer

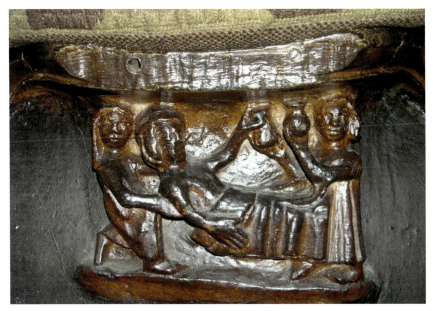

Figure 4: A sick man supported by a woman, while a doctor looks at two flasks in his hands. Misericord at Great Malvern Priory St Mary and St Michael's, Worcestershire.

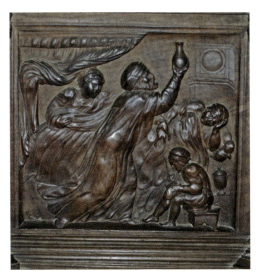

Figure 5: A doctor-uroscopist, carved on a panel of the choir stalls of the cathedral in Sevilla.

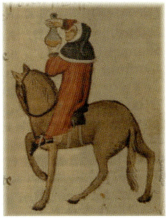

Figure 6: Even when on horseback, the uroscopist was able to make a diagnosis! Ellesmere manuscript, c.1420, Huntington Library, San Marino, California.

monkeys simultaneously "ape" the inadequacy of physicians, remind viewers of the need to care for the health of their souls on earth and sometimes seem to be looking through or beyond the glass to the spiritual salvation that only the Church could provide. Foxes dressed as preachers remind audiences against the dangers of false preachers, who are not what they seem. Perhaps apes were also used to represent the medical profession because they were prone to self-adoration and grooming (the sin of vanity!).[4]

Ape-physicians are frequently found not only in manuscripts, (Figs. 7,8,9 and 10) but also in carvings and even on stained glass in the borders of an early 14th century window at York Minster. (Figs. 11 and 12) The misericord carvings of circa 1520 in Beverley Minster and St Mary's, for example, depict a wide variety of animal activities, including the preaching fox and a bagpipe-playing sow, along with a number of scenes involving apes.

At Boston, St Botolph's in Boston in Lincolnshire, a late 14th century misericord shows a fox consulting an ape doctor. (Fig. 13) The latter inspects the flask, whilst the fox holds what has been suggested as a bucket containing a sample of droppings,[4] but we believe this is the typical bag in woven straw used to protect the matula.

In the Church of St Anne in Knowle, Warwickshire, the ape, who wears a monk's cape, lectures to the fox while pointing at the flask in his hand. (Fig. 14) Horst Janson[6] notes that representations of ape-physicians begin to appear in the 14th century.

6
Janson H.W., *Apes and Ape Lore in the Middle Ages and the Renaissance*, p.168, London, 1952.

On a choir stall in Cologne Cathedral an ape-physician with a matula is anointing an owl, a creature of the night, and therefore associated with the forces of darkness. (Fig. 15) The association of an ape, without a matula and an owl, also occurs in the misericords of the cathedrals in Winchester (Fig. 16) and Toledo (Fig. 17).

Physicians caricaturised as apes are also found in English misericords at Bristol, Cartmel, Manchester, Westminster Abbey in London, St Stephen's Church at Sneiton in Nottingham, and in Norwich. (Figs. 18-23, respectively). In St Mary's Church in Beverley, Yorkshire there are two misericords dating from c.1445, with apes as uroscopists. One misericord (Fig. 24) shows a wildman (or "woodwose") with a bow and arrow, hunting a fox. The fox is wounded and is holding out a bag of money to an ape that is chained up. The ape is holding a flask of urine. Another misericord in the same church (Fig. 25) shows a scene that has been interpreted as one in which the ape offers his services to a wealthy man - probably a cleric - who holds a large coin - marked with a cross - whilst shunning the other figure.

Christa Grössinger[7] however, suggests that the item raised by the figure on the left is not a coin but, rather, the Eucharistic Host. And Paul Hardwick[8] writes: *The object to which our ape-physician addresses himself, then, could be both Host and, as the poem "Salve lux mundi" puts it, "journey-money for our pilgrimage" through this life and into the next.*

We must remember that by the mid 15th century the significance of the Eucharist had caused it to become one of the most controver-

---

[7]
Grössinger, C. *The World Upside-Down: English Misericords*. 101. Harvey Miller: London, 1997.

[8]
Hardwick, P. "A problematic representation of the Eucharist in Beverley St Mary's," in: *The Profane Art of the Middle Ages*. 11, 159-173, 2003.

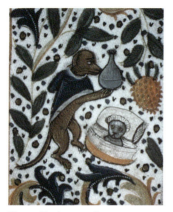
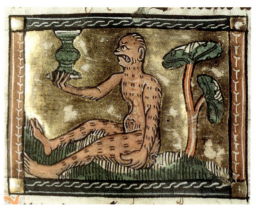

Figure 7: An ape-doctor examines the urine of a child-ape. The Mac Kinney Collection of Medieval Medical Illustrations, University Library, Edinburgh, D.b3.20, folio 25v.

Figure 8: A naked ape as a uroscopist! Der Naturen Bloeme, c.1350, Kon. Bibl. The Hague, KB, KA 16.

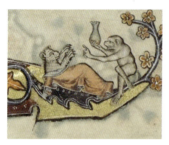

Figure 9: An ape-doctor examining the urine of a sick bear (?). Macclesfield Psalter, Fitzwilliam Museum, Cambridge.

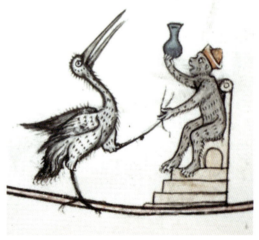

Figure 10: An ape-doctor examining the urine of a heron and feeling its pulse. Pontificale of Metz, 1316, Fitzwilliam Museum, Cambridge, 298, folio 81r.

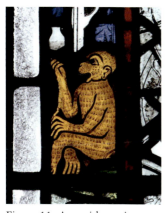

Figure 11: Ape with a urine flask, stained glass window, York Minster.

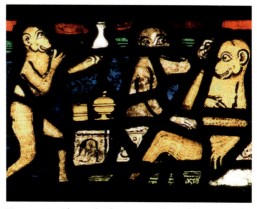

Figure 12: Along the lower margins of the stained glass of a window, in a manner comparable to the borders of an illuminated manuscript, animals and birds parody human behaviour in York Minster. A monkey doctor examines a urine flask, while a sick ape is attended by a monkey-doctor.

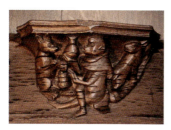

Figure 13: At St Botolph's Church in Boston in Lincolnshire, a late 14th century misericord shows a fox consulting an ape doctor.

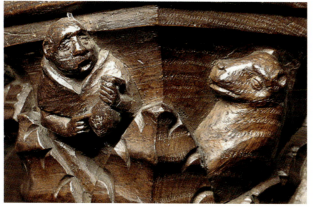

Figure 14: In the Church of St Anne, Knowle, Warwickshire, the ape, who wears a monk's cape, lectures to a fox, while pointing at the flask in his hand.

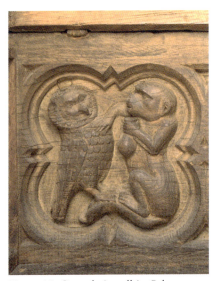

Figure 15: On a choir stall in Cologne Cathedral an ape-physician with a matula is anointing an owl, a creature of the night, and therefore associated with the forces of darkness.

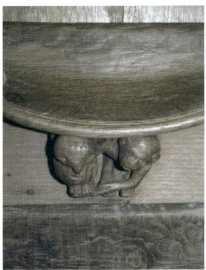

Figure 16: The association of an ape, without a matula and an owl, also occurs in the misericords of the cathedral in Winchester.

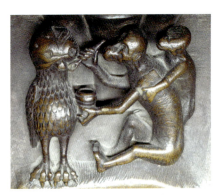

Figure 17: Another association of a ape-doctor and an owl in the cathedral at Toledo.

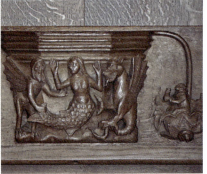

Figure 18: Misericord in Bristol Cathedral. On the right side stands a naked ape with a monk-cape and a matula in his hands. Notice also the symbolic mermaid with two devils.

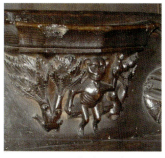

Figure 19: A naked monkey holding up a urine bottle, as a satirical jibe at the little respected medical profession. Misericord in the Cartmel Priory Church of St Mary and St Michael, Grange-over-Sands, Cumbria, dated 1440.

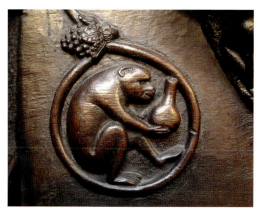

Figure 20: On the misericords in Manchester Cathedral, we can see two ape-doctors on the lateral sides of a misericord. One ape is looking at a urine flask, the other is holding a child.

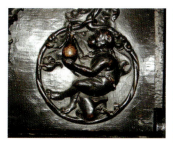

Figure 21: Ape examining a matula. Misericord in the collegiate church of St Peter, Westminster Abbey, London.

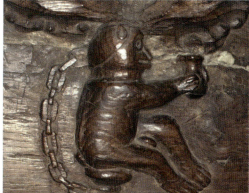

Figure 22: Naked and chained ape looking at an urine flask. St Stephen's Church, Sneiton, Nottingham.

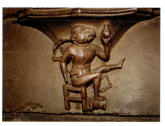

Figure 23: Naked and chained ape-doctor examining a matula. Misericord in St Andrew's Church, Norwich.

sial elements of doctrine in the English Church, because in the late 1370s Wyclif had rejected the doctrine of transubstantiation, instead arguing that the bread and wine remained materially unchanged by consecration, although the spiritual being of Christ also became present.

The Church of St. Mary, at Bury St. Edmunds, Suffolk, was first constructed circa 1110-20, but was rebuilt between 1425-30. It contains some of the finest woodwork to have survived the vandalism of Cromwell. The roof can be dated to 1430-1440. One of the most interesting features about these wood-carvings is that a number of them have some relationship to disease or medicine. Bury St. Edmunds has long been an important medieval centre for infirmaries.[9]

[9] Rowe J., *The medieval hospitals of Bury St. Edmunds*, Med. Hist., p.253-63, 2, 1958.

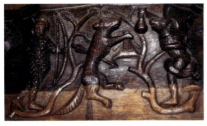

Figure 24: In St Mary's Church, Beverley, Yorkshire, a misericord shows a wildman or woodwose with a bow and arrow hunting a fox. The fox is wounded and is holding out a bag of money to an ape that is chained up. The ape is holding a flask of urine (partly restored).

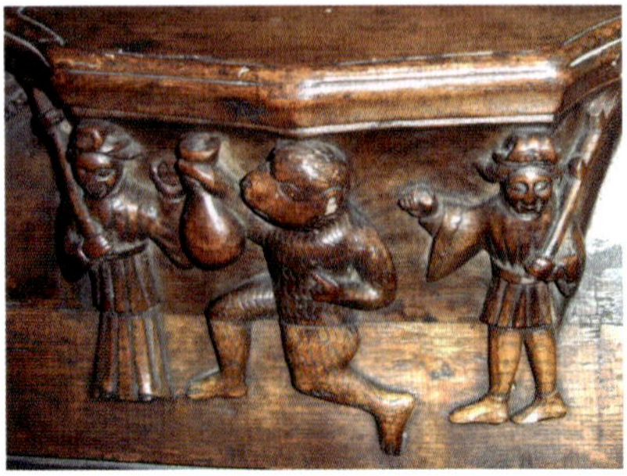

Figure 25: Another misericord in St Mary's shows a scene that has been interpreted as an ape offering his services to a wealthy man – probably a cleric – who holds a large coin – marked with a cross - whilst shunning the other figure. This might not be a coin but the Eucharistic Host. The figure at the right could be a bell ringer (partly restored).

It catered not only for the medical needs of its own monastic and secular population but also for the vast numbers of pilgrims. On the roof of the church there are six carvings related to uroscopy. One carving shows a doctor with his matula. It is interesting to see that, apart from his hat, the doctor appears naked, an unusual depiction for this period. A single snake climbing around a staff can be seen in front of the dog. (Figs. 26 and 27)

Another carving in the same Church shows a monkey with collar and chain holding a urine flask. The physician is again caricaturised as an ape.[10]

In the St Mary of Charity church in Faversham, Kent, an ape chained to a clog and holding an upturned flask is carved on a misericord. (Fig. 28)

Throughout its history, the parodic animal physician has always invoked laughter. The very audacity of the image suggests the *inversus mundi* in several ways. First, there is the absurdity of depicting an animal engaging in one of the most complex human arts. A second element of the parody lies in showing an animal caring for the physical health of its traditional nemesis. This second aspect goes beyond mere humour and invokes widespread suspicion of the physician-patient relationship. And so D.A. Sprunger writes[5]: *thus the image of the parody animal-physician reminds us that truth can lie not at the center of things but at the edges.*

Surviving literary texts certainly attest to this 'suspicion of the physician-patient relationship'. One of the most lively satires of the quack

---

[10] Wells Calvin, *Fifteenth-century wood-carvings in St. Mary's Church, Bury St.Edmunds*, Med. Hist. 9,(3): p.286-88, July 1965.

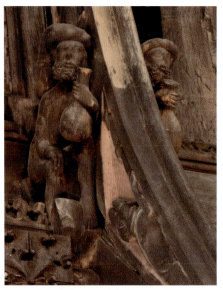 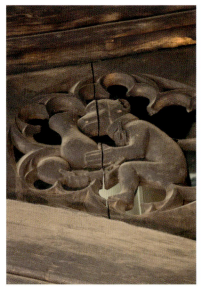

Figure 26: A doctor with his matula. The doctor appears naked, an unusual depiction for this period. A single snake climbing around a staff can be seen in front of the dog. Woodcarving, St Mary's Church, Bury St Edmunds, Suffolk.
©Photo Ricky Wilkinson.

Figure 27: Another carving in St Mary's shows a monkey with collar and chain holding a urine flask.
©Photo Ricky Wilkinson.

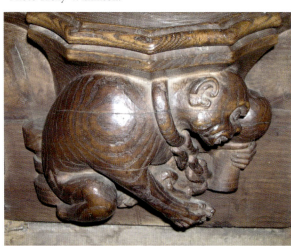

Figure 28: Misericord in the St Mary of Charity Church, Faversham, Kent. A fat ape chained to a clog, holding an upturned and empty urine flask.

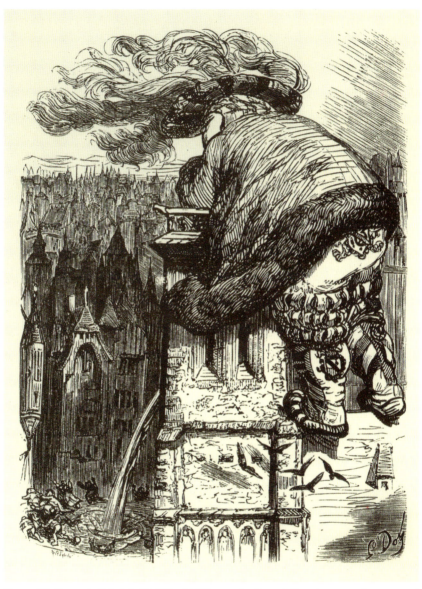

Figure 29: François Rabelais (?1494 - 1553), a major French Renaissance writer, created such fictional characters as Gargantua and Pantagruel, who were giants travelling around the world. Gargantua is said to have urinated on Parisians, (*compissant les parisiens*) over Notre-Dame Cathedral.

doctor appears in *The Simonie*, a vigorous attack on the abuses of the times, which ran to three versions in the second and third quarters of the 14th century:

Another craft Y se also that towcheth the clergie:
that be this fals fisicianes that helpeth men to die.
They wil wagge the vryne and vrynal of glas
And suere that he is sikerer than euer yit he was
And sayn,
'Dame, fore defaute of help, Thyn hosbonde is ney slayn.'

After 'wagging the urine', he goes on to fleece the wife, force an evil concoction down the hapless patient and take the best of the food for himself, before concluding his business:

'Dame,' he seith, 'drede the noght, the maister is wonne,'
And likket.
But thus he bereth awey the siluer and the wif beskikket.[11]

Urinating

In medieval iconography, urinating men are frequently seen. Even in places we wouldn't normally expect: churches and official buildings. In daily language and humour, the act of urination was not as obscene as it is today!

François Rabelais (1494?-1553), a major French Renaissance writer, and also a medical doctor created fictional characters such as Gargantua and Pantagruel, who were giants travelling around the world. Gargantua is said to have urinated on Parisians, (*compissant les parisiens*) over the Notre-Dame. He took away the bell from the Cathedral and humourously explained the origin of the name 'Paris' (English translation, from Chapter 1, Section XVII):

[11] Hardwick Paul, *Through a Glass, Darkly: Interpreting Animal Physicians*, Reinardus, Vol. 15, n°1, p.63-70, John Benjamins Publishing Company, 2002.

And they pressed so hard upon him that he was constrained to rest himself upon the towers of Our Lady's Church. At which place, seeing so many about him, he said with a loud voice, 'I believe that these buzzards will have me to pay them here my welcome hither, and my Proficiat. It is but good reason. I will now give them their wine, but it shall be only in sport.' Then smiling, he untied his fair braguette, and drawing out his mentul into the open air, he so bitterly all-to-bepissed them, that he drowned two hundred and sixty thousand, four hundred and eighteen (260,418), besides the women and little children. Some, nevertheless, of the company escaped this piss-flood by mere speed of foot, who, when they were at the higher end of the university, sweating, coughing, spitting, and out of breath, they began to swear and curse, some in good hot earnest, and others in jest. Carimari, carimara: golynoly, golynolo. By my sweet Sanctess, we are washed in sport, a sport truly to laugh at; in French, "Par ris", for which that city hath been ever since called Paris; whose name formerly was Leucotia, as Strabo testifieth, lib. quarto, from the Greek word Greek, whiteness,-because of the white thighs of the ladies of that place. (Fig. 29)

As we already mentioned, the iconography on misericords often describes popular tales but also popular proverbs. The proverb *piss against the moon*, was one such well-known saying. Perhaps the best-known painting of this proverb is one of the *Twelve Proverbs* painted by Pieter Brueghel the Older (1525-1569) in 1558. (Fig. 30) The same painter illustrated the same proverb on another of his masterpieces: *Flemish Proverbs or The Reversed World*. In this

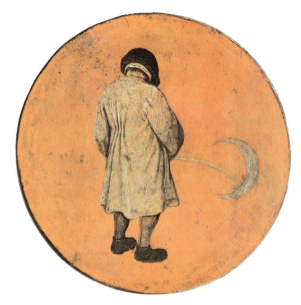

Figure 30: *Pissing against the moon*, painting of the Flemish proverb by Pieter Brueghel, 1558. Museum Mayer van den Bergh, Antwerp.

1559 painting a man is pissing through an open window against a flag with a crescent moon. Frans Hogenberg (1535-1590) also produced an etching, *Die Blauwe Huycke,* in which a man is also urinating against the moon.[12]

One of the explanations of this proverb in Dutch is: *Wat ick vervolghe, en geraecke daer niet aen. Ick pisse altyt tegen de maen*. (Whatever I do, I never attain my goal. I am always pissing against the moon = my great ambitions are without success).

Jan Grauls[13] does not agree with this meaning of 'to try the impossible' and he argues that the proverb instead describes someone who is unhappy and whose dealings brought him only constant concern. On the other hand, B. van de Walle concludes in his very interesting article[12]

12
Van de Walle, B. "Pisser contre la lune: imprudence insolence ou quête de l'impossible," in: *Incontinences urinaires de l'homme*, by R.J. Opsomer & J. de Leval. Springer, 2011.

13
Grauls Jan, *Volkstaal en volksleven in het werk van Pieter Brueghel*, p.210, NV Standaard Boekhandel, Antwerp-Amsterdam, 1957

that *pissing against the moon* might indeed mean to *try the impossible*, and *he pissed against the moon* could signify that he only attracted misfortune.

A French dictionary by Rey and Chantreau[14] mentions that "pissing against the sun" means: *s'en prendre aux puissant, être insolent* (to bring the powerful on one's self, to be insolent). In St Martin's Church in Bolswaard, The Netherlands, a damaged misericord also illustrates a man pissing on the world. (Fig. 31)

One of the 54 misericords in the collegial church of Saint-Martin-de-Champeaux, made in 1522 by Maistre Richard Falaise, shows a man pissing with a good stream of urine into a winnow. (Fig. 32) Art historians have always explained this woodcut as an illustration of the French proverb *petite pluie abat grand vent* (small rains calm big winds) but Jan Grauls[13] suggests that the winnow should be identified as a radiant against which the man is pissing and should therefore be seen as an illustration of the proverb *pissing against the sun*!

A misericord in the 'Grote Kerk' at Breda, The Netherlands, shows a man, drinking from a big jug and urinating into a receptacle. (Fig. 33) This is also the illustration of an old Dutch proverb: *die veel drinkt, moet ook veel pissen* (whoever drinks a lot also has to piss a lot!). On a misericord in the St Materne Church in Walcourt, Belgium, a man is urinating from a distance into a big jar held by a woman. (Fig. 34)

Urinating men are not only found in churches of that period but also on civil buildings such as a urinating woman on the town hall in St Quentin, France. (Fig. 35) On top of the

14
Rey A., Chantreau S., *Dictionnaire des Expressions et Locutions*, Les Usuels du Robert, Paris, 1982.

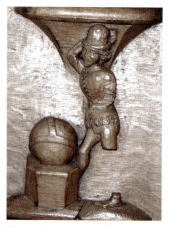
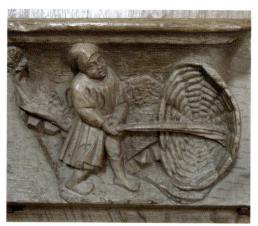

Figure 31: *Pissing on the world*: a Dutch expression carved in the wood of a damaged misericord. St Materne Church in Bolswaard, The Netherlands.

Figure 32: One of the 54 misericords in the collegial church of Saint-Martin-de-Champeaux, made in 1522 by Maistre Richard Falaise, shows a man pissing with a good stream of urine into a winnow.
©Johan J. Mattelaer

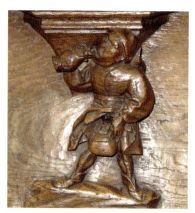
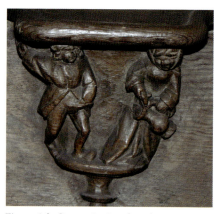

Figure 33: A misericord in the 'Grote Kerk' at Breda, The Netherlands, shows a man drinking from a big jug and urinating into a receptacle. This is also the illustration of an old Dutch proverb: *die veel drinkt, moet ook veel pissen* (whoever drinks a lot also has to piss a lot!). © Johan J. Mattelaer

Figure 34: On a misericord at the St.-Materne church in Walcourt, Belgium, a man is urinating from a distance into a big jar held by a woman.
© Johan J. Mattelaer

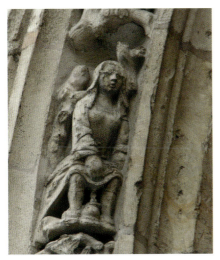

Figure 35: Lady, urinating into a piss-pot. Carving on the town hall in St.-Quentin.
© Johan J. Mattelaer

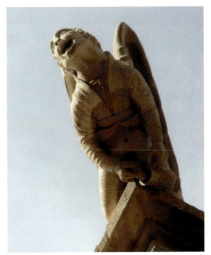

Figure 36: An angel pissing in a receptacle on top of the Lonja de Mercaderes in Valencia.

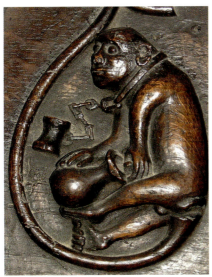

Figure 37: An ape urinating into a matula on a misericord in the Holy Trinity Church in Stratford-on-Avon.
© Giles C. Watson.

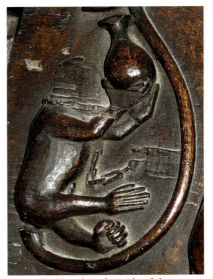

Figure 38: On the other side of the same misericord a (decapitated) ape examines the matula.
© Giles C. Watson

Lonja de Mercaderes in Valencia an angel, pissing into a receptacle can also be seen. (Fig. 36)

Urinating ape-doctors

An ape urinating or staring into a matula is also a satire on quack doctors, who set great store by the colour and opacity of their patients' urine as a means of diagnosis.

We find an ape urinating into a matula on one of the misericords in the Holy Trinity Church in Stratford-on-Avon. (Fig. 37) At the other side of the same misericord a (decapitated) ape examines the matula. (Fig. 38) The iconography of an ape urinating into a matula inspired Giles C. Watson to write the following poem in 2011:

The ape-doctor prognosticates his own ruin
The pee's the thing, wherein
I'll scry my own prognosis:
I dare not blench, but I
Must face it: thrombosis,
Embolism, imbalance
Of one or other humour,
Spasms, syphilis,
Some tumid tumour -
Besides which, I have lately
Quaffed ale, and not a little:
So I must needs die of pain
Or otherwise take a pittle.
The question is not
Ontological:
To pee, or not to pee?
The answer's logical:
I need not fear the bite
Of spider, or of adder:
The biggest risk's
An impacted bladder.

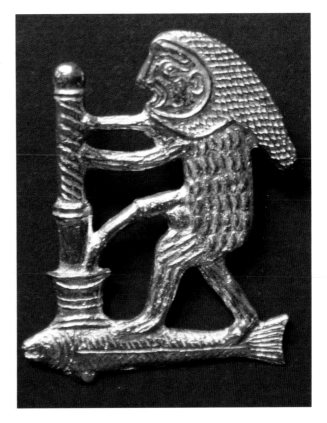

Figure 39:
Ape urinating into a mortar, insignia found at Salisbury, England, 15th century. Replica by Lionheart Replicas.

In medieval times, from 1250 to 1550, pilgrimages were extremely popular all over Europe. St. James of Compostela, in Galicia (Spain) was one of the most popular destinations. Pilgrims wore special insignia, in an alloy of tin and lead, on their clothes or attached to their staff, because anyone bearing such an insignia could count on the hospitality of the local people. The cheap insignia were also worn to protect the wearer from the evil eye and to bring good luck. In Salisbury, England, an insignia was found that depicts an ape as a physician, grinding medicine in a mortar and pestle, to which he adds his own urine. (Fig. 39)

The Church despised doctors in favour of the miracle working powers of shrines. As such, this badge may very well be an example of Church propaganda.

Conclusion

In medieval times, uroscopy was the main diagnostic tool for medical doctors. The urine flask or matula became the symbol of medicine. However, the practice was open to abuse by unscrupulous physicians, who offered treatment solely on the basis of uroscopy, without even seeing the patient. Although more orthodox practitioners and physicians tried hard to distance themselves from the practice, by the 15th century the art of uroscopy was falling into disrepute and the matula became a symbol of ridicule. On the carved misericords in choir stalls, the physician holding a matula was commonly represented as an ape-doctor, with the allegorical implications of foolishness, vanity and even lechery.

Correspondence to:
Dr. J.J. Mattelaer
Albijn van den Abeelelaan12
8500 Kortrijk – Belgium
johan.mattelaer@skynet.be

FROM *"DEVIL'S TEMPTATION"* TO *"EROTIC IMAGINATION"*

Sergio Musitelli[1], Ilaria Bossi [2]

1. Expert of the EAU History Office.

2. MD University of Milan – Internal Medicine II – HL Sacco (Italy)

Athanasius, Bishop of Alexandria (295-373 AD), gave the first and detailed account of the so-called *Temptations of St. Anthony* in his *Life of St. Anthony*, written either about 357 A.D., or – according to some historians – between 365 and 373AD. Before 388 AD, Evagrius of Antioch († after 392 AD) translated Athanasius' work into Latin and the tradition of the *Temptations of St. Anthony* would exert a strong and fundamental influence not only on Christian doctrine, but also on the art of both Western and Eastern Christianity in the subsequent centuries. This influence would be felt until at least the second half of the 17th century.

Obviously, they thought that the devil, or rather a sort of demons' Sabbath, was the cause of these "temptations" – most probably based on the *Temptations of Our Lord Jesus Christ* in the desert, described by the Gospels of *Matthew* (4, 1-11), *Marc* (1, 12-13) and *Luke* (4, 1-13) – and countless painters represented the *Temptations of St. Anthony* as the effects of the black arts.

Suffice it to confine ourselves to observing some of the most famous paintings like Martin Schongauer's (1435-1491) engraving (Fig. 1), Hieronymus Bosch's (1450-1516) painting (Fig. 2) or Mathis Grünewald's (1460-1528) painting (Fig. 3) to have the clearest idea of such "demonic" interpretation of the *Temptations*.

By contrast, the Galilean scientific revolution, according to which the basis of knowledge is the "sensata esperienza", .i.e. the "sensible experience", was accepted by the whole European culture and mainly by the English, Flemish and French cultures. Firstly, this caused the English philosophical empiricism, founded by John Locke (1632-1704) and increased and perfected first by the genius of Isaac Newton (1642-1727) under the scientific, then by David Hume (1711-1776) from a philosophical point of view. In addition, it was Hume's work which paved the way for modern psychology and, consequently, for the modern psychoanalysis and psychiatry.

Étienne Bonnot de Condillac (1715-1780), in his turn, developed philosophical empiricism into "sensualism" and paved the way for the future "positivism" we shall deal with below.

At any rate, these new and revolutionary ideas influenced both literature and art. With regards to literature, suffice it to quote Daniel De Foe's (1660-1721) and Jonathan Swift's (1667-1745) novels and to compare them with the medieval ones to understand the difference perfectly. As for the arts, the new empirical cultural climate suggested a new perception of the so-called *Temptations of St. Anthony to the painters*, the first example of which –as far as we know- is David Teniers the Younger's (1610-1690) painting. (Fig. 4)

As one can see, the painter has confined the demons to secondary particulars, whilst the real protagonists of the "temptations" are human figures that confront the Saint.

Everyone knows that the English *"empiricism"* and the consequent French *"sensualism"* paved the way for the positivistic reaction against Georg Wilhelm Friedrich Hegel's (1770-1831) "absolute idealism". Positivism was founded by August Comte's (1798-1857) *"Cours de philosophie positive"* (1630-1842) and, on its turn, influenced not only science – suffice it to remember the fundamental contributions of Jacob Molesschotte (1827-1893) and Ivan Petrovič Pavlov (1849-1936) – but also both literature and art.

As for Literature, suffice it to quote Honoré de Balzac's (1799-1850), Émile Zola's (1846-1902) novels and mainly Gustave Flaubert's (1821-1880) *"Les Tentation de Saint Antoine"* (1849, but published posthumously in 1910).

However, positivism influenced mainly the arts in general, and painting in particular: the *Temptations* become clearly the result of "erotic imagination" as many pictures prove, starting from Theodore Chassériau's (1819-1857) *"Temptations of St. Anthony"* (Fig. 5) to pass to Domenico Morelli's (1826-1901) *"Temptations"* (Fig. 6) where provocative female nudes have replaced the traditional tempting demons. This *"erotic"* perception of the *"temptations"* reached its peak in Paul Cezanne's (1839-1906) paintings (Figs. 7 and 8) and in the painting of Lovis Corinth (1858-1925). (Fig. 9)

However, it is exceptionally interesting to observe that this desecrating interpretation of the *"temptations"* as an effect of *"erotic imaginatio*n" goes back to the 14th century. Indeed, one can easily find it already represented by the

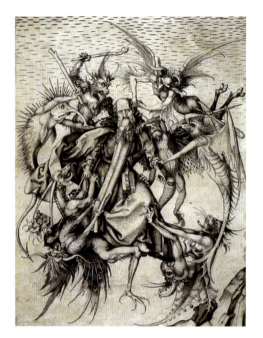

Figure 1:
New York Metropolitan Museum of Art.

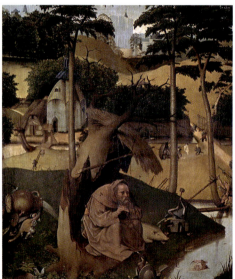

Figure 2: Madrid, Museo del Prado.

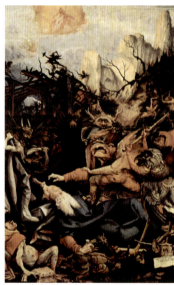

Figure 3: Colmar, Schongauer Museum in the Unterlinden Monastery.

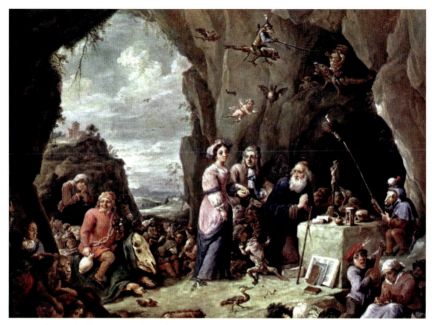

Figure 4: Madrid, Museo del Prado.

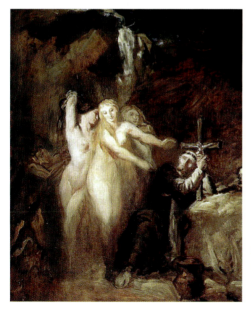

Figure 5:
Paris, Musée d'Orsay.

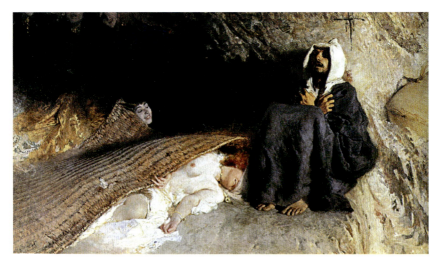

Figure 6: Rome, Galleria Nazionale d'Arte moderna.

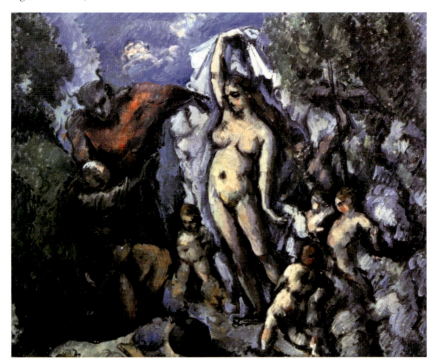

Figure 7: Paris, Musée d'Orsay.

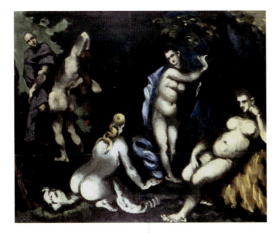

Figure 8:
E.G. Buhrle collection (Switzerland).

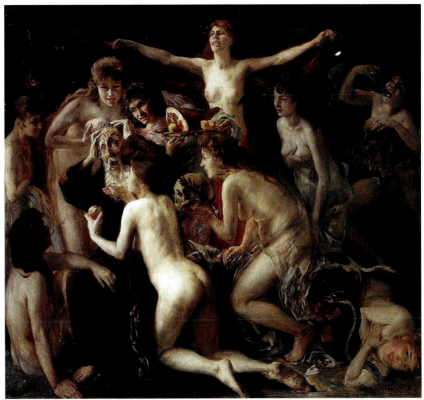

Figure 9: Bern, Kunstmuseum

unconventional genius of Giovanni Boccaccio (1313-1375). In the 10th novella of the 3rd day of his *Decameron*, Dionaeus – who is really Boccaccio himself – tells the story of how *"Alibech becomes a hermit, whom the hermit Rusticus teaches to put the devil into hell."*

The events happen as follows: Alibech is a very beautiful 14 year-old girl, the daughter of a rich man and she lives in Capsa, Egypt. She is not Christian, but, having heard that to serve the Lord is the most beautiful thing, and that the wisest servers stayed in the desert, she decides to reach them in order to learn how to practice the service. After a very long walk, she meets an old hermit and tells him the reason of her trip. The old hermit fears that she is the devil himself in disguise of a beautiful girl.

However, the legitimate suspicion arises that Boccaccio's words have two meanings. Indeed, he writes *"temendo non il diavolo lo ingannasse"* which may mean "fearing that the devil would deceive him" as well as "fearing that his penis would betray him", i.e. "would not have any erection", because, in the story, as we shall see, the "devil" is just the penis! At any rate, he refreshes her and tells her that not far from his own shack there is a much wiser hermit, who will teach her much better. Alibech thanks him, moves and reaches the second hermit, who gives her the same answer and sends her to a further one. He is Rusticus, a young ascetic, who "wants to make a great trial of his saint determination." He welcomes her and prepares a pallet for her.

However, the temptations "began fighting against his strengths, which were much feebler than he supposed and took flight in a moment", so that he began studying how he could obtain what he wanted without letting Alibech understand that "he fancied her as a debauchee". As he realized that she had not yet had any sexual intercourse, he informed her that "the most terrible enemy of the Lord was the devil", that "the best and most pleasing service to the Lord was to put the devil into the hell, where He had condemned him" and that she had to behave like him in order to serve the Lord at best.

At this point, he undressed himself. Obviously, the girl too undressed herself. This done, it resulted in "the resurrection of the body", as Boccaccio elegantly and ...religiously calls the penile erection. Alibech sees this strange and still unfamiliar phenomenon and asks Rusticus: "Rusticus, tell me: which is that thing that protrudes so much, and I have not it?" and he answers: "Dearest girl, it is just the devil, you are right, but you have another thing that I have not...You have the hell!". Alibech puts herself at Rusticus' disposal and agrees that he must put the devil into hell. At first she suffers from a certain pain owing to defloration, and: "No doubt – she tells – this devil is a very bad thing and a real enemy of our Lord, because even in hell, let alone when he stays out of it, he causes pains when he is there!"

However, she soon begins taking a great delight in "serving the Lord" and pushes Rusticus repeatedly to go on casting the devil into hell telling him: "Rusticus, I do not succeed in understanding why the devil flees from hell, because should he stay in the hell as gladly as the hell receives and keeps him, he would never leave!" This being the fact, in the course of time she complains with Rusticus: "If your devil – she tells him – has been punished enough and does not trouble you any more, my hell torments me!" However, Rusticus, "who fed himself exclusively on roots and water", could not satisfy her as she wanted.

At last, a fire destroyed the house of Alibech's father and killed the whole family, so that Alibech was forced to leave Rusticus and to go back to Capsa to prevent the properties from being seized. When back in the city, the women asked her what she had done in the desert. Alibech told them that she had served the Lord, described how she had performed the service, and caused general belly laughs: she could perform such a service at best also in Capsa with the aid of Aderbale, who would marry her!

Apart from the fact that we would today charge Rusticus with paedophilia (Alibech is only fourteen years old!), Boccaccio's story is exceptionally interesting under the psychological and sexological point of view. Let us deal first with Alibech: the pains caused by defloration and the subsequent and ever increasing pleasure she feels in "*putting the devil into the hell*" are an exceedingly right and correct statement!

As for Rusticus, we must point out the following series of observations. Although we wonder how many "*Alibechs*" Boccacio knew before beginning the undertaking of his "*Decameron*", nonetheless he has surely given us an "*ante litteram*" or brief treatise on sexual anthropology. There cannot be any doubt that a certain amount of gynaecophobia is present in the story of Alibech and Rusticus and that it was most probably suggested by the biblical

Figure 10: Rome, St. Mary of the Victory.

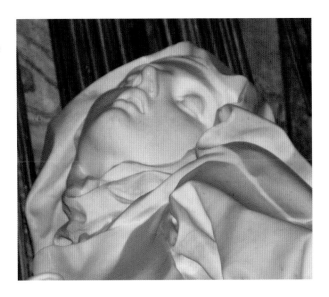

Liber Tobiae. However, misogyny joins with the strength of sexuality, which acts like a sort of Aristotelian *"motionless mover"*. Under this sexological point of view, we can emphasize some fundamental elements that Boccacio raises:

1) Deprivation of food in general, and of proteins in particular (Rusticus *"fed himself exclusively on roots and water"*!) may cause not only sensory hallucinations, as well as spark of *"erotic imagination"* (as Hildegard of Bingen's (1098-1179) and Teresa of Avila's (1515-1582) writings prove), but also erectile dysfunction, as the behaviour of the first anchorite seems to allude to. Gianlorenzo Bernini (1508-1680), in his turn, represented realistically and rather unscrupulously the *"Ecstasy of Saint Teresa"* as an orgasm, rather than as a mystical ecstasy. (Fig. 10)
2) Rusticus' *"iuvenilis redundantia"* is surely the effect of an excess of testosterone, and overcomes every spiritual and mystical ambi-

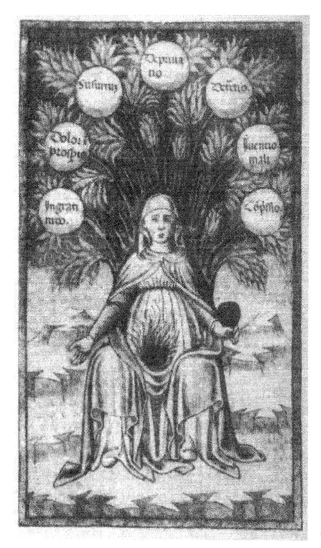

Figure 11:
Woman as the "source of all evils" in a miniature of the 15th century.

tion, most probably after having suffered from a lot of pollutions, although Boccaccio does not point out this particular.

3) As for the repeated sexual intercourses, they concern not only the male *"mythology"* of as many as possible intercourses, but also the female nymphomania, which is often anorgasmic, although this does not seem to be the case of Alibech. At any rate the failure of erection, which Rusticus suffers from after so many copulations, does not need any particular comment, because it was an as normal phenomenon at Boccaccio's time, as it is nowadays.

4) Finally, we must observe that the perception of the woman as a *"sexual object"* pervades Boccaccio's view. He did not know the role of the amygdala as the brain centre of both fear and pleasure, this is true, but he anticipated the contradiction – which characterizes the subsequent century – between voluptuousness – extolled by Lorenzo Valla's (1407-1457) *"De voluptate"* (On pleasure) – and the *"woman source of all evils"* as was still represented in many manuscript illuminations till the end of the 15th century. (Fig.11)

Correspondence to:
Prof. Dr. Sergio Musitelli
20080 ZIBIDO SAN GIACOMO (Mi) – Italy
S.S. dei Giovi n. 69
Phone: +39-029053748
Fax: +39-029053748
E-mail: sergio_musitelli@alice.it

DEPICTION OF VENEREAL DISEASES ON WAX MODELS IN THE MOULAGE MUSEUMS OF PARIS AND ATHENS

E. Poulakou-Rebelakou[1], M. Karamanou[1], A. Rempelakos[2] and G. Androutsos[1]

1. Department of History of Medicine, Athens University Medical School, Athens, Greece.

2. Urologic Department "Hippocrateion" Hospital, Athens, Greece.

Introduction

The illustration of venereal diseases with the use of wax models in a realistic three-dimensional representation far surpassed any other available teaching aid, such as the two-dimensional paintings and photographs, from 18th century until the 1950s. At that point, colour photographs replaced moulages in the study of venereology and dermatology.

The creation of the first dermatologic moulages is credited to Franz Heinrich Martens (1778-1805) of Jena, Germany. As a physician and medical illustrator, he published in 1804 an Atlas of venereal diseases and started making venereological moulages until his untimely death, a year later. Only six of his moulages have survived in the Jena Anatomic Institute Museum. The true pioneer, however, is Joseph Towne (1806-1879) who worked all his life as a medical illustrator and moulager at Guy's Hospital in London. A third wax modeler, Anton Elfinger (1821-1864) worked for the dermatologist Ferdinand von Hebra to cast dermatologic moulages for the department at Vienna.[1]

These first physician-artists paved the way for the rise of dermato-venereologic moulage which gradually -with the increase of scientific communication in the second half of 19th

1
Joshi, R. "Moulages in dermatology-venereology". *Indian J Venereol Leprol*. 2010. 76 (4): 434-38.

century- passed into international acceptance as a very effective model for teaching medical students.

The Parisian and the Viennese traditions

In the second half of the 19th century, Paris and Vienna became centres for the institutionalisation of the young field of dermatovenereology and at the same time also developed important moulaging tradition.[2]

2 Schnalke, T. "A brief history of the dermatologic moulage in Europe. Part III Prosperity and decline". *Int J Dermatol.* 1993. 32: 453–63.

In Paris, the tradition of moulage making started in the Hospital of St Louis, when the professor Charles Lailler (1828-1898) met the artist Jules Baretta (1834-1923) who was producing papier-mâché models of fruit in the Passage Jouffroy in Paris.[3] (Fig.1)

3 Schnalke, T. *Diseases in Wax: The History of the Medical Moulage.* Quintessence: Chicago, 1995. 85-91, 93-101.

Working in the Hospital of St Louis in Paris, Baretta created his first moulage in 1865 and by the time he died he had sculpted about 2000 wax moulages depicting skin diseases. His creations were renowned for their extraordinary detail. However, in the same way as his English colleague Joseph Towne, Baretta did not reveal the secrets of the technique he used. Professor George Photinos, in 1907, gave the standard interpretation of this taciturnity over the subject: "Before the mouleurs reach perfection, they have to invest effort and time. They have to learn two things. First, they need to gain at least basic knowledge in dermatology and venereology. Second, they have to invent some kind of method to produce the casts. The consequence was that until recent years no mouleur was willing to share his technique with another for fear of no longer being able to make a living from his art, if someone else learned from him".[4]

4 Photinos, G. "Die Herstellung und Bedeutung der Moulagen (farbige Wachsabdrücke)". *Dermatol Z.* 1907. 14: 131–157.

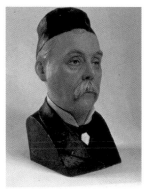
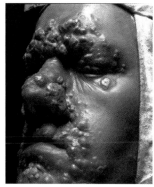

Figure 1: The eminent mouleur Jules Baretta. Wax bust from the museum of St. Louis Hospital in Paris.

Figure 2: A moulage from the museum of St. Louis Hospital in Paris, demonstrating lesions of secondary syphilis of the face.

The mouleurs' silence had also other dimensions which were rooted in the special setting they created with their patients to form good moulages: an atmosphere of openness, trust and credibility. It was the distinguished mouleuge Elsbeth Stoiber (1924-) who broke the taboo of secrecy and explained the details of moulage production. She explains that the mouleur had initially to touch the sick person while he applied the modeling material to the body. In the following meetings, he would paint and prepare the moulage in a realistic way in order to create a correct replica of isolated bodily structures in the context of a "true portrait" of a sick individual.[5]

Baretta's astonishing moulages were first presented in 1889, August 5-10, during the 1st International Congress of Dermatology and Syphilology, held in Paris. (Fig.2) Some of the Congress attendees, impressed by the artistic and scientific result of the moulage display,

---

5
De Chadarevian S. and N. Hopwood. *Models: the third dimension of science*. Stanford University Press: Stanford, 2004. 225-229.

decided to create similar collections in their own departments. Nowadays, the moulage collection of the Hospital St Louis is the largest in the world and the total stock includes 4000 items.

The Vienna moulage tradition was established by Moritz Kaposi (1837-1902), son-in-law of Hebra, after his return from Paris and the aforementioned Congress of 1889. He appointed Carl Henning (1860-1917), a physician and medical illustrator, to work on a wax collection that was greatly admired in 1892 during the 2nd International Congress of Dermatology and Syphilology, held in Vienna. After Henning's death in 1917, the moulage-making was taken over by his son Theodor, so that father and son dominated the field in Vienna for more than half century. The Vienna collection includes 3000 moulages and is the second largest in the world.[4]

The moulage museum of Andreas Syngros hospital in Athens

Moulage-making spread to many countries and had also reached Greece. In Athens, the Andreas Sygros Hospital was founded in 1910, as a dermato-venereological hospital. Its first director and first University Professor for dermatology and syphilology, George Photinos (1876-1958), created a museum of wax models in 1912. (Fig.3)

Photinos was trained in Paris (1902-1905), Berlin, London and Vienna and kept constant and close contact with scientists from all over Europe. However, his main scientific orientation and inspiration was Paris and he had the dynamic and creative temperament to organise the new hospital, despite the adverse political situation then reigning in Greece (The Greek-Turkish and Balkan Wars).

Photinos was exposed to the moulage technique both in Paris and especially in Berlin, by the moulager Heinrich Kasten at the clinic of Oskar Lassar. The initial wax models of the Athens collection (today the third largest international collection after Paris and Vienna) are credited to have been made by Photinos himself. (Fig.4) [6]

Later, the moulages were produced by specially trained craftsmen such as the painter Constantine Mitropoulos, a graduate of the Athens School of Fine Arts (1892). After him, the art of moulage-making passed on to his son George, who was, according to the older employees of the hospital, an even greater artist, passionate with his job. It is broadly accepted that the Greek moulages are of an artistic quality, easily recognised.[7] (Fig.5)

Three items from Athens representing syphilis (with the signature of the artist Constantine Mitropoulos) have been donated to Paris' museum and sixty items to Paris' Military School Val de Grace at the request of Dr Arnaud, presenting frostbite modelled on the soldiers of the siege of Bizani (Ioannina) during the Balkan Wars (1912-1913). Twelve moulages were donated to Professor Photinos by the staff of the Parisian Hôpital du Midi.[7]

The cultural treasures of the moulages collection consisting of 1660 items depicting a variety of skin diseases are exhibited in wooden showcases furnished with crystal doors and divided into two large rooms with 29 and 34

---

[6]
Hadjivassiliou, M., A. Katsambas and A.M. Worm. "The Greek Moulages: A picture of skin diseases in former times". *J Eur Acad Dermatol Venereol.* 2007. 21: 515-519.

[7]
Emmanouil, P.E. "Museum of wax models," in: *Museum of Moulages of "Andreas Sygros Hospital,"* A. Katsambas, P. Emmanouil and T. Petridis. (eds.). MD Publications: Athens, 2006. 9-15.

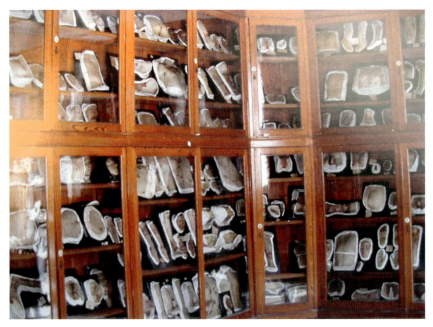

Figure 3: Part of the moulages exhibition from the museum of Moulages of "Andreas Sygros" Hospital.

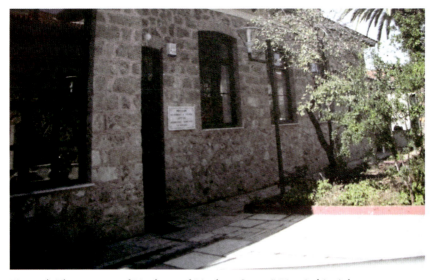

Figure 4: The museum of Moulages of "Andreas Sygros" Hospital in Athens.

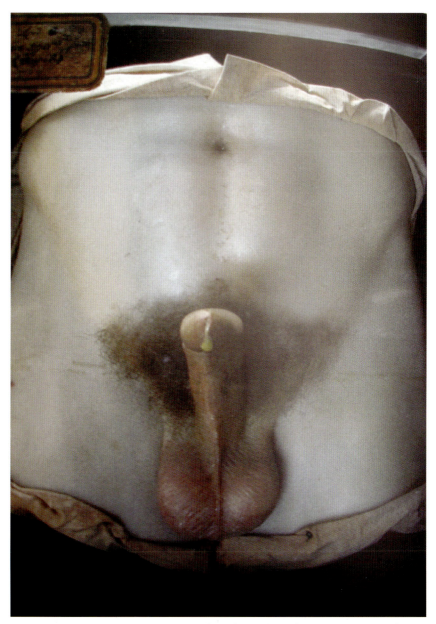

Figure 5: A moulage from the museum of Moulages of "Andreas Sygros" Hospital, representing a urethral discharge.

showcases respectively. An antechamber contains 12 display-cases. Among the wax models, several represent genitalia. In Athens, as in Paris, the collection includes the more intimate parts of the body and these moulages were produced applied on the nude human body, especially the suffering body.[7]

Conclusion

In their own way, it was the patients that contributed to the advancement of medical knowledge, through their close and trusting collaboration with the hospital's physicians and artists. The creation of a wax model demands the close collaboration of at least three people: the patient with the specific disorder, a doctor for the diagnosis and a cast craftsman capable of reproducing the full details of the disease so that optimal results may be obtained both in the creation and the reservation of the wax model.

Correspondence to:
Marianna Karamanou, M.D
4 str. Themidos, Kifissia
14564, Athens, Greece
Tel: +30 697 3606804
Fax :+30 2108235710
E-mail: mariannakaramanou@yahoo.com

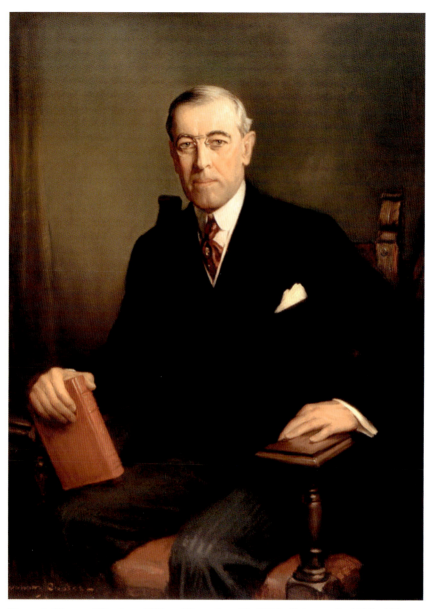

Figure 1. Thomas Woodrow Wilson (December 28, 1856 - February 3, 1924), 28th President of the United States. Married Edith Bolling Galt in 1915, despite objections from his advisors that remarriage could cost him the re-election.

PRESIDENT WILSON AND THE MANAGEMENT OF URINARY RETENTION A CENTURY AGO

Jennifer Gordetsky[1], Ronald Rabinowitz[2]

1. University of Rochester, Department of Pathology

2. University of Rochester, Departments of Urology and Pediatrics

In October, 1919, President Woodrow Wilson suffered a stroke, leaving him paralysed on the left side. During the acute phase of his recovery, the President suffered from urinary retention, which led to a urologic consultation for its management. In this article, we will discuss the case of President Wilson's urinary retention and the standard management of this urological condition in 1919.

Thomas Woodrow Wilson (December 28, 1856 - February 3, 1924) was the 28th President of the United States. He received a baccalaureate degree in 1879 from Princeton University and a doctorate in American history, economics, and government from Johns Hopkins University in 1885.[1] In 1902 Wilson became the President of Princeton University and went on to become the Governor of New Jersey in 1910. Wilson won the presidential election of 1912 when William Howard Taft and Theodore Roosevelt split the Republican vote.

A literature search was performed on the management of President Wilson's urinary retention and the different treatments of urinary retention, including cystotomy and suprapubic prostatectomy between 1889 and 1926.

Straight catheterization

President Wilson's urinary retention was initially managed with straight catheterization.

1

Texter, J.H. "The President's Dilemma: 1919". *Va Med Q* 1980; 107: 757-762.

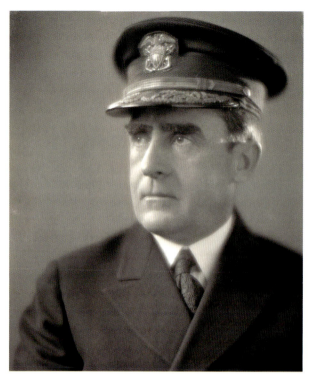

Figure 2: Admiral Cary Grayson. Per Mrs. Wilson, Grayson advised against surgery because he did not believe her husband could survive the operation.

After a few days, passing a catheter per urethra became impossible. A discussion was held as to whether to pursue a suprapubic cystotomy. Surgical intervention was declined or refused due to the President's poor health. In 1919, similar cases of urinary retention due to prostatic hypertrophy were often treated with suprapubic cystotomy followed by immediate or delayed prostatectomy. In the most experienced hands, the overall mortality associated with the operation was 5.5%, and reported as high as 25% in the literature. Urinary retention treated by intermittent catheterisation had a mortality rate up to 80%, due to urinary tract infection. The decision of how to manage the President's urinary retention was a difficult one.

The President's condition

The year was 1919, World War I had just ended, and President Thomas Woodrow Wilson was in his second term of office. Wilson had suffered multiple illnesses throughout his life. He had poor vision from measles since childhood, suffered a spontaneous retinal haemorrhage at age 37, and a retinal detachment when he was 48. In addition, he also reportedly had recurrent, severe headaches and issues with indigestion. On April 13, 1919, the President suffered a severe febrile illness, with coughing and diarrhoea, thought to be a case of influenza.[1]

Although he recovered, the President looked grey and tired and was noted to have marked twitching of his facial muscles.[2] On September 3, 1919 the President began a trip across the nation to campaign for joining the League of Nations. Due to Wilson's poor health, the trip was strongly discouraged by his physician, Rear Admiral Cary T. Grayson. Wilson delivered 32 major addresses over a period of 22 days. During this time, he suffered from severe headaches, double vision, and difficulty breathing, requiring him to sleep in a sitting position.[1-3]

These signs suggested cerebral vascular insufficiency and cardiac failure. The trip was abruptly ended on September 25, 1919, when Wilson suffered a stroke while giving a speech at Pueblo, Colorado.[1,2] He lost vision, had left-sided facial paresis, and difficulty speaking.[1,2] By the time the President returned to Washington several days later, his condition had improved and he was able to walk unassisted.[1,2] According to Grayson, "On the evening of October 1st he seemed quite bright and cheerful, played bil-

2
Weinstein, E.A. *Woodrow Wilson: A Medical and Psychological Biography*. Princeton University Press: Princeton, 1981. 349-359.

3
Grayson, C.T. *Woodrow Wilson: An Intimate Memoir*. Holt Rinehart and Winston: New York, 1960. 96-110.

liards a few minutes, and appeared better than any time since he started on the western trip. But then early the next morning the crash came."[3]

At 8:00 am, October 2, 1919, President Wilson suffered a severe stroke, with left hemiparesis. During the first few days Wilson's condition was guarded and several physicians were consulted by Grayson including Doctor Charles Mayo.[3] The President's condition slowly improved, but almost two weeks later he began having difficulty voiding. Since the Foley catheter would not be invented until 1934, Admiral Grayson performed straight catheterization, which he found to be difficult.[4]

The President's urinary retention continued and the following day Grayson was unable to pass a catheter. Dr. H. A. Fowler was called and, after trying multiple instruments, was able to finally empty the bladder.[4] A day later, on October 17, straight catheterization again became necessary and neither Grayson nor Fowler were able to pass a catheter. Dr. Hugh Young, Chief of Urology at Johns Hopkins, was consulted. At this time the President had gone thirty hours without voiding and his abdomen was described as being "hugely distended"[4].

A discussion was held on whether to proceed with surgical intervention. According to Dr. Young's autobiography, he considered performing a suprapubic cystotomy but did not think the President could tolerate the procedure in his condition. He believed that the obstruction would eventually be forced open by the internal pressure in the bladder and therefore recommended waiting.[4]

4
Young, H.H. *Hugh Young: A Surgeon's Autobiography*. Harcourt Brace and Company: New York, 1940. 398-403.

Apparently Dr. Young and Dr. Fowler took a drive around Washington while they waited for the President's urinary retention to resolve on its own.[4] During this trip they purchased several urologic instruments that had yet to be tried on the President.[4] According to Dr. Young, by the time they returned the President had voided spontaneously.[4]

The First Lady

According to Edith Galt Wilson, the President's wife and a direct descendant of Pocahontas, the events regarding management differed substantially compared to Dr. Young's recollection.[5] She stated that Dr. Fowler and Dr. Young had decided that there was no alternative but an operation. Dr. Grayson did not feel the President could handle the stress of surgery and left the decision of whether to operate to Mrs. Wilson. She decided against surgical intervention, stating that "Nature will finally take care of things, and we will wait."[5]

At this point she said that Dr. Young followed her into her dressing room and proceeded to draw diagrams and continued to argue in favour of surgery saying, "You do understand, Mrs. Wilson, the whole body will become poisoned if this condition lasts an hour, or at the most two hours, longer."[5] Despite his attempts, she stayed fast in her decision to withhold surgery.

Treatment of urinary retention in the early 20th century

Urinary retention remains one of the most common conditions that urologists treat today. Nowadays, urinary retention is easily managed with the use of indwelling catheters,

---

[5] Wilson, E.B. *My Memoir*. The Bobbs-Merrill Company: New York, 1938. 291-292.

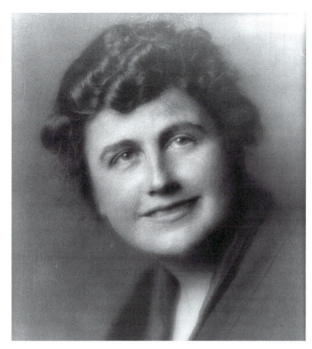

Figure 3:
Edith Bolling Galt Wilson. Descendant of Pocahontas, Martha Washington, and Thomas Jefferson. In Edith's autobiography she claimed that Dr. Young recommended surgery, which she refused.

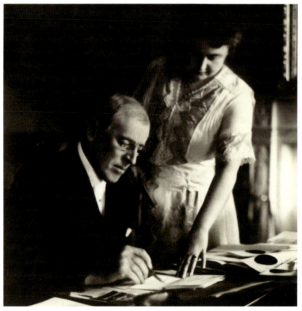

Figure 4.
During Wilson's incapacity, Edith was instrumental in the management of the President's health and political affairs. In this photograph she holds a paper steady for her husband to sign.

alpha-adrenergic blockers, 5α-reductase inhibitors, and transurethral resection of the prostate by either traditional or laser techniques. Antibiotics have made death from urinary sepsis a rare complication. But in 1919, urinary retention was a serious urologic condition with a significant mortality rate.[6]

In fact, the management of urinary retention in cases of spinal cord injury during World War I had been referred to as "one of the surgical failures of the war".[6] At the King George Military Hospital from May 1915 to the end of 1916 there were 339 cases of spinal cord injury with bladder function involvement. Of these men, 160 died from urinary tract infection (47% mortality) during the first 8-10 weeks following injury. In 1919, the mortality due to urinary sepsis in spinal cord injured patients was 80%.[6]

The principal reason for this high mortality rate was that intermittent straight catheterization was the treatment of choice for urinary retention. Due to the lack of sterile technique and antibiotic therapy, urinary tract infection was almost inevitable, estimated at 90% of cases, and sepsis often followed shortly thereafter.[6]

Some surgeons made the argument that mortality would be reduced by performing an early suprapubic cystotomy followed by placement of a self-retaining or sewn-in catheter.[6,7] Cystitis, they argued, could be managed through bladder washing, and since the bladder was no longer under pressure, sepsis was much less common.

Bladder massage was another method of treating urinary retention. The bladder was

---

6

Thomson-Walker, J. "The treatment of the bladder in spinal injuries in war." *Br J Urol* 1937; 9: 217-230.

7

Hoffman, J. "The rationale and Technique of Supra-pubic cystotomy." *Proceedings of the Philadelphia County Medical Society*. 1891; 12: 358-364.

gently but firmly compressed and massaged through the abdominal wall with the object of expressing urine. This was repeated every 4-6 hours. Some reported this method to be very successful in at least partially emptying the bladder while others reported difficulty due to contraction of the bladder neck and urethral sphincter.[6] This technique, when successful, prevented the need for catheterisation, however bladder rupture had been reported.[6]

In 1891, hypertrophy of the prostate was regarded as a "hopeless condition, both from a medical and surgical standpoint."[7] Around 1900 came the description of the suprapubic prostatectomy as a treatment for prostatic hypertrophy. Eugene Fuller is accepted by most historians as the originator of the idea of suprapubic prostatectomy. However, Peter Freyer is given credit for making this surgical approach popular through multiple publications including detailed case reports.

By 1919, suprapubic cystotomy followed by either immediate or delayed prostatic enucleation was successfully used as treatment for this "hopeless condition." In 1919, the mortality of the procedure was reported in the literature to be as high as 25%.[8] Though the most experienced surgeons reported a mortality rate as low as 5% and an operative time of 3 to 8 minutes.[8,9] In *Young's Practice of Urology*, published in 1926, the mortality for prostatectomy is reported as high as 25%. However, Young stated that with the proper preoperative treatment (drainage of the bladder, management of infection, correction of kidney function, etc) the mortality was reduced "to practically zero."[10] He reported a mortality of 2-3% for suprapubic

8
Milford, H. "Prostatectomy, Suprapubic and Perineal". *Medical Science Abstracts and Review*. 1919: 420-432.

9
Freyer, P.J. "Total enucleation of the Prostate: A Further Series of 550 Cases of the Operation." Brit Med J. 1919: 121-125.

10
Young, H.H. and D. Melvin. Davis, and Franklin P. Johnson: *Young's Practice of Urology*. Vol. 1. W.B. Saunders: Philadelphia & London, 1926.

drainage alone, which he said was "a mortality probably higher than prostatectomy itself."

Young also reported a series of 1,049 consecutive cases of perineal prostatectomy up to October 15, 1922, with an overall mortality of 3.4%. Interestingly, the mortality declined from 8.4% in 1903 to 2.4% in 1919. Although the mortality for prostatectomy was high, the mortality from urinary sepsis was much higher. However, given the President's guarded condition, the management of his urinary retention was a difficult decision.

Conclusion

President Wilson's urinary retention after his stroke was thought to be as a result of his immobility and enlarged prostate. In 1919 the options for urinary retention included watchful waiting, straight catheterization, and suprapubic or perineal cystotomy followed by immediate or delayed prostatectomy. Regardless of who made the decision, due to the risks of surgery the President was ultimately treated with watchful waiting. His urinary retention improved over the next several days and he became incontinent of urine for the next few weeks. This resolved and within a few months normal voiding returned.[1]

Correspondence to:
Jennifer Gordetsky
Jennifer_Gordetsky@urmc.rochester.edu
601 Elmwood Avenue, Box 626
Rochester, NY 14642
585-797-5759
Fax: 585-273-3637

THE DISCOVERY OF AN EARLY 13TH CENTURY FRAGMENT OF GILLES DE CORBEIL'S *CARMINA DE URINARUM IUDICIIS*

Evelien Hauwaerts[1], Johan R. Boelaert[2]

1. Ph.D., researcher at the medieval manuscripts department at the Public Library of Bruges, Belgium.

2. M.D., unit of nephrology and infectious diseases, Algemeen Ziekenhuis Sint-Jan, Brugge, Belgium. Now retired.

During the general cataloguing campaign of medieval manuscripts of the Bruges Public Library, a fragment of the *Carmina urinarum iudiciis* by Gilles de Corbeil was discovered. The hitherto unnoticed fragment of the *Carmina* is comprised of one sheet, or folio, that is part of the binding of the Bruges Public Library, Manuscript 230. This manuscript dates from the 14th century and is more recent than the fragment itself, which probably dates from the first half of the 13th century. In the Middle Ages, the parchment of older, obsolete books was often recycled to strengthen the binding of new books. This is also the case here. The parchment folio with the fragment of the *Carmina* was used by the bookbinder to protect the book block of manuscript 230 from the wooden plates or covers. The folio was possibly pasted on the inner side of the plate pastedown, or was inserted as a supplementary sheet in-between the book block and the wooden plate (fly leaf or end leaf).* (Fig. 1)

* The original binding of ms. 230 was replaced over the course of the history. Its current binding is a modern conservation binding of leather on cardboard plates. On the verso of the folio, the imprint of a previous (perhaps the original) leather binding is still clearly visible.

** For a description of MS 230, see the Brugge Openbare Bibliotheek's digital catalogue at: http://cabrio.bibliotheek.brugge.be/erfgoed/.

The text on the sheet which was used, was irrelevant to the bookbinder. The strength of the parchment on which the text was written was what mattered. The contents of the fragment also bear no relation to the content of manuscript 230, which contains the sermons of Johannes de Friburgo (circa 1250-1314).**

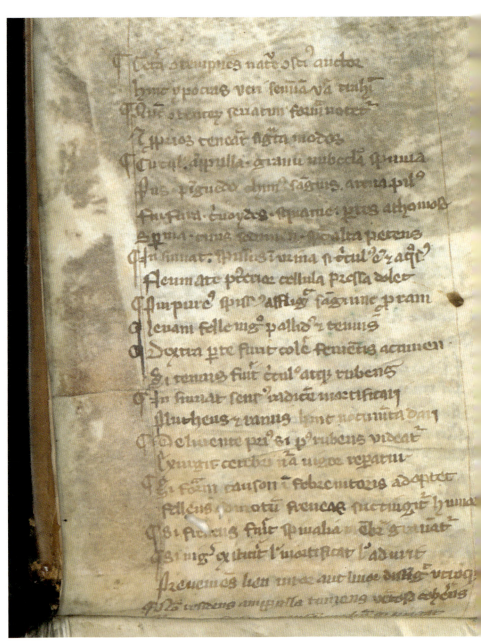

Figure 1: Bruges, Public Library, Ms. 230, fly leaf recto.

¶ Splenē si nimiis radiis iugata coruscet.
¶ Siccū monstrat epar effusio larga liquoris.
¶ Insolite anuua si moribi limine talis.
Precipitando malum sine vernicia liquoris.
¶ Infrenco frenesim notat. ¶ sub fine duelli.
Designat orcior fmari sidera paris.
¶ Fleumaos et cole que sacro muie reddit.
Crenam tenuē atrū semnius humor.
¶ Distans obscure tenuis tiena humoris.
In muliere notat motus metas eclipsim.
¶ Plus tenue acrius tenue qm nimis rescidue
¶ Intensam cū febre mag. sine febre remissa.
¶ In rufum ingens puri color enuit āia
Equalis purus medius cui se liquor uiuit
Corporis erratia ualidos denunciat actus.
¶ In puero iuuene seue fleumatico mulie.
Bufa udues tenuis notat k incommoda febs
Acuuia treu duplicē. ¶ sed tempore longo
Epatis offensam ut febrem quatridianam
¶ Principio cause dū sit noua semina morbi.
Bufa pax tenuis aluis summū regionem.
Nubes rara tenes morbi gnata calons.
  De salso propriā succendi fleumata febrem
¶ Sed crevm mocho una gradente agnure.
¶ Spissa pur um non crevm maiōtruosam

The fragment of the *Carmina* covers the recto and verso side of the fly leaf, each in two columns.* It starts with *'Et sine febre fuerit enormes excitat actus'* and ends with *'Principio cause dum sunt nona semina morbid rufa parum tenuis cuius'*.** From the style and writing (a gothic *textualis libraria*) it can be deduced that the fragment of the *Carmina* probably dates from the first half of the 13th century. Since the *Carmina* was probably written before 1193 (see below) and the author Gilles de Corbeil died around 1220, this is an early copy in the *Carmina* text tradition. Whenever a new edition of this text will be issued, it will certainly have to take account of this fragment.

The most recent edition, drafted by Camille Vieillard, dates back to 1903.*** The fact that the corpus of sources is incomplete warrants a new edition. There are about ten of other known 13th-century copies of this work, or fragments of this work, but there is no precise dating of these copies. A thorough examination of the stemma [genealogy] or text pedigree of the *Carmina* is necessary to place the Bruges copy among the other copies in terms of chronology and text purity.****

Gilles de Corbeil

Not much is known about the life of Gilles de Corbeil, also called Aegidius Corboliensis. We can only guess his date of birth; he died around 1220. However, it is certain that he was born in Corbeil in the French department of Marne, that he followed medical studies in Salerno, Southern Italy, and that he was among the first professors to lecture in medicine in Paris –he was perhaps even the first[1]. He was appointed as chief physician (archiater) by the

* In fact this concerns a bifolium or double sheet. The folding line and the holes which the sewing thread passed through in the binding which has been undone, that is to say the binding from which this folio was taken for recycling, are still visible. The sheet is 22 cm long along the outer side and is 14 cm wide along the upper side (i.e. according to the current binding).

** The text begins at the top of column a on the verso side (26 visible lines), and continues in column b on the verso side (idem), then column a on the recto side (25 visible lines) and in column b on the recto side (idem).

*** Camille Vieillard, *L'urologie et les médecins urologues dans la médecine ancienne. Gilles de Corbeil, sa vie, ses oeuvres, son poème des urines*, Paris: F. de Rudeval, 1903.

**** The oldest copy does not necessarily contain the text which is closest to the author's original. A newer copy from a less corrupted branch of the genealogy can contain a "purer" version than an older copy and therefore take precedence in a possible edition.

[1] Ausécache, M. "Gilles de Corbeil ou le médecin pédagogue au tournant des 12ième et 13ième siècles." *Early science and medicine*. 3 (1998) 190.

French king Philip-August and he was canon of Notre-Dame in Paris.

Gilles's training in Salerno was a very significantly defining point in his life. This Southern Italian city was, particularly between the 11th and 13th centuries, a *civitas Hippocratica*, an intellectual hotbed where many practitioners and scholars, especially laymen, with particular interest in medicine, wrote books and gave instructions and took care of the sick. Salerno formed a bridge between the Greek, Latin, Jewish and Arab worlds.

A key figure was the medical scholar Constantinus Africanus (1015-1082), born in Carthage or Kairouan (in modern Tunisia), who spoke Greek, Arabic and Latin fluently and had travelled through the Middle East. In the Benedictine Abbey of Monte Cassino, near Salerno, he focused on translating medical treatises. He translated the available Arabic translations of the Greek texts of Hippocrates and Galenus to Latin and translated the Arabic works of his predecessors such as Isaac Judaeus (also known as Isaac Israeli, circa 880 – circa 955), and the Persian Haly Abbas (circa 925 – circa 994).

This important translation work offered the Salerno school the opportunity to study the works of the greatest scholars of antiquity in depth and to become acquainted with the Arab contribution to medicine. The absorption process of these translations by Constantinus Africanus bore fruit in the mid-12th century: in Salerno numerous writings appeared which studied medical theory more in depth than the previous, more empirically oriented works from this city.

For several centuries they then remained as standard works in use.² Here we cite only the most important: a small collection of medical texts mainly from antiquity, which would constitute the basis of medical didactic education and would later bear the name *Articella* or minor art; the *Regimen sanitatis Salernitanum*, a general work on health education that spans the centuries; the *Glossae* or commentary by Matthaeus Platearius (d. 1161) on the *Antidotarium* of Nicolaus of Salerno, a basic work on herb preparations; the *Circa instans*, presumably by the same Platearius, a botanical work concerning simple herbs which also introduced Eastern herbs; the commentary of four Salerno masters on the *Practica chirurgiae* of Roger of Frugardo (end of the 12th century); and finally the *De mulierum passionibus* or *Liber Trotula*, a work on gynaecology that is attributed to the female author Trota and of which the Bruges Public Library has a 15th-century Middle Dutch translation.*

2 Pasca, M. "The Salerno school of medicine." *American Journal of Nephrology*. 14 (1994) 480.

Inspired by his education in Salerno and full of praise for his teachers, Gilles taught the Salerno medical theories in the burgeoning Paris university, using his own writings. He left us five works.³ Three medical works were written before 1193: *Carmina de urinarum iudiciis, Liber de pulsibus metrice compositus* and *De laudibus et virtutibus compositorum medicaminum*. From a later date are *Viaticus signis et symptomatibus aegritudinum*, which has survived only partially, and a non-medical work titled *Hierapigra ad purgandos praelatos*, a satire against the abuses of the high clergy. We limit our discussion to the first three works which have survived in full, with a particular focus on the *Carmina de urinarum iudiciis*, further abbreviated as *Carmina*, of which an old fragment has been discovered in the specified Bruges fly leaf.

3 Vieillard, C. *L'urologie et les médecins urologues dans la medicine ancienne: Gilles de Corbeil; sa vie, ses oeuvres, son poème des urines*. Paris, 1903. 209-65.

* A full file on this manuscript and its translation (with scans, edition, articles) is available online via: www.historischebronnenbrugge.be.

The texts

As their respective titles indicate, both the *Carmina* as the *Liber de pulsibus metrice compositus* are written in verse. This also applies to Gilles's two other medical writings: the botanical poem about the *composita* or compound medicines and the book on pathology. Medical writings in verse were not new: Avicenna (980 - 1037) had written the medical treatise *Canticum*, better known as *Canon*, in poetic form.

In Salerno however most medical texts - except for the *Regimen sanitatis* - were prose. This was particularly the case with the Salerno sources of direct inspiration of Gilles' *Carmina:* the *Tractatus de urinis* and the *Regulae urinarum* of Maurus and the *Compendium de urinis* of Urso.[4] Gilles explains the reason he opted for verse in the introductions of his urine poem and his pulse poem: "What is intended for memory, is better entrusted to a short verse than to cumbersome prose." His intention was twofold: he attempted to give his writings an aesthetic character and to promote the memory process of his students.

The theories Gilles proposes in his *Carmina* reflect the state of knowledge of the time concerning the origin of urine and on the application and utility of uroscopy. Very briefly summarised, uroscopy in antiquity served to determine the prognosis, but it was not meant to indicate the disease of a specific organ. A major turning point was expressed in *De urinis*, written by the Byzantine Theophilus (possibly in the 7th century).[5,6] For the first time, this author quite rightly defined the origin of urine in percolation (filtration) of the blood - only the blood, not the humors or elemental fluids of the body - in the kidneys. He developed a method of urinalysis

---

[4] Pasca, 481.

[5] Angeletti, L.R. and B. Cavarra. "Critical and historical approach to Theophilus' De Urinis." *American Journal of Nephrology*. 14 (1994) 285-87.

[6] Wallis, F. *Acta Hispanica ad Medicinae Scientiarumque Historicam Illustrandam*. 20 (2000) 38-57.

that focused on the amount of urine, its density, colour and sediment. He distinguished ten colour shades for "light" and ten for "heavy" urine.

His urinalysis not only indicated a specific prognosis but also diseases of certain organs or feverish illnesses. These new insights by Theophilus were partly taken up by Isaac Judaeus and became accessible in Salerno through the translation work of Constantinus Africanus. Isaac, the Salerno scholars and, in their wake, Gilles embraced Theophilus's theory that urine is formed in the kidney by percolation. They believed, however, that it was a percolation not only of blood but also of humors. Uroscopy would mainly provide information about the condition of the liver, from which the humors originate, and the urinary tract.

Gilles' *Carmina* begins with a short introduction in prose, the poem that follows consists of two parts and an epilogue. In the first part urine is described as follows:

> *Sanguinis est urina serum, subtile liquamen*
> *Humororum, quos conficit ars regitiva secundi*
> *Et princeps operis...*
> (Urine is the serum of the blood, the subtle residue
> of the humors, arising from the force which drives
> the second digestion...)

According to the prevalent pathophysiological scheme at the time, a first digestion of food took place in the stomach, a second – as mentioned in the cited verses - in the liver, and a third in the blood vessels. The poem continues with a detailed description of the colour nuances that

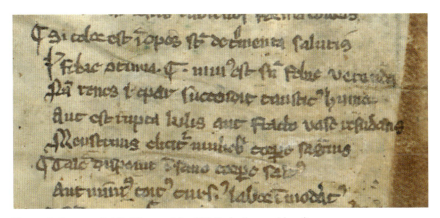

Figure 2: Bruges, Public Library, Ms. 230 fly leaf verso (detail).

[7] Moulinier-Brogi, L. "L'uroscopie au Moyen Age." *Lire dans un verre la nature de l'homme.* 2012, Editions Champion, Paris. 145.

urine can adopt, with their respective meanings. For Gilles, there were twenty important colours, for his predecessor Maurus, there were nineteen.[7] We cite an example from the fly leaf (Fig. 2):

Si color est inops sunt detrimenta salutis
In febre continua minus est sine febre verenda
Nam renes uel epar succendit causticus humor
Aut est rupta kilis aut vase resudans
Menstruus elicitur muliebri corpore sanguis
Talem disponit in sano corpore saltus
aut nimius coitus cursus labor immoderatus.
(If the {urine} colour resembles that of old wine, it is a bad sign
with continuous fever; in the absence of fever that colour is to be feared less
and it springs from a humor which heats the kidneys or liver,
or a rupture of the portal vein or {another} vein or from menstrual blood.
In healthy humans dancing, excessive sexual intercourse, walking,
or excessive labour can trigger {that urine color also}).

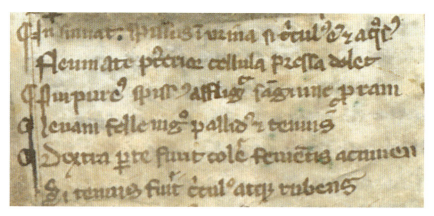

Figure 3: Bruges, Public Library, Ms. 230 fly leaf recto a column (detail).

These verses illustrate the concept that the colour of the urine reflects the state of the humors (bodily fluids). A certain dyscrasia or imbalance between the four humors can result in the heating of certain organs, which in turn results itself in a specific urinary color. The last two verses urge caution with physical excesses, which is fully in line with what is proclaimed in the *Regimen sanitatis*, which was created in Salerno a few generations before Gilles' residence there. Further in his poem Gilles states that urine sometimes arranges itself in three layers: an upper, middle and lower. Each urine layer then refers to a corresponding part of the body. Therefore urine functions as a sign or signature. According to this conceptual framework, later called the signature theory, characteristics for example, of plants and in our case of urine, correspond to parts of the human body, which emphasises the unity of divine creation.

The second part of the *Carmina* presents the importance of nineteen constituents which can be found in urine. In the epilogue, the poet commemorates his teachers in Salerno. To illustrate the second part we have selected a passage from the fly leaf, in which Gilles explains the first of nineteen constituents of urine, namely the circle. This is the most superficial layer of the urine that takes a circular shape in the matula (urine glass).[8] (Fig. 3):

[8] Veillard, 76-78.

> *Insinuat spissus in vrina si circulus est et aquosus*
> *Fleumatfurit colere feruentis acumen*
> *Si tenuis fuerit cie posterior cellula pressa dolet*
> *Purpureus spissus affligit sanguine proram*
> *Leuam felle nigro pallidus et tenuis*
> *Dextra parte furit colere feruentis acumen*
> *Si tenuis fuerit circulus atque rubeus*
> (A thick watery circle on the urine
> Indicates suffering in the posterior part of the head under pressure of the phlegm.
> A thick red [circle indicates that] the blood is affecting the prosencephalon.
> A pale and thin [circle signifies] suffering in the left hemisphere under the influence of black bile.
> In the case of a red and thin circle hot yellow bile is raging on the right side of the head.)

The humoral theory is ubiquitous in this passage. Each of the four humors is responsible, not only for certain characteristics in uroscopy, but also, and more importantly, for specific disease patterns. These last verses do not hesitate in presenting an extensive anatomical localisation of the suffering.

In summary, the analysis of both the colour and the *contenta* of urine, discloses not only the interaction between the humours, but also offers an insight into a particular diagnostic direction.

Gilles's second poem, *Liber de pulsibus*, begins with an explanation in prose about human physiology. The four main organs are the brain, seat of sensation and motor function, the heart, seat of vegetative functions and breathing, the liver, seat of body nutrition and growth, and the testes, seat of multiplication. The basic body is the liver, and the other main organ is the heart. Urine primarily reflects the condition of the liver and the urinary tract, while the pulse presents the condition of the heart. Hence the predominance of the urinary and pulse examination for diagnosis. The poem deals with three aspects of pulse analysis: the ten pulse variants with components, detection of the pulse and the theory of pulse signs.

Gilles's third poem, *De laudibus et virtutibus compositorum medicaminum*, is an adaptation in verse of the commentaries of Matthaeus Platearius on the antidotarium of Nicolaus. Gilles selects 80 of the 140 compounds dealt with by Platearius. He does not repeat their preparation formulas, but he extensively praises the power and scope of application of these preparations.

Conclusion

What is the historical importance of Gilles de Corbeil? He was one of the great Salerno figures who, through their research into the formation, the colour and the constituents of urine, contributed to a better understanding of the physical world and sought connections between elements, bodily fluids, colours and disease.[9]

[9] Moulinier-Brogi L. 166.

Through his writings the medical intellectual heritage that had been consolidated in Salerno thrived in Paris and from there radiated to Northern Europe. It was a type of medieval learning that had arisen in a secular environment and was naturalistic, more deeply rooted in Greco-Roman and Arabic medical learning than in biblical or ecclesiastical considerations. Gilles is situated at the transition from oral teaching, as in Salerno, to a university education of students. He has contributed to the institutionalisation of medical education, which in turn promoted the professionalisation of the medical profession. His classes were supported by a written treatise, his choice of verse facilitated memorization.

In any case, Gilles's poetry was particularly praised throughout the late Middle Ages. This is testified by the numerous copies of his *Carmina*, whether or not provisioned with commentaries by leading physicians including Gilbert Anglicus (circa 1180 - circa 1250), Bernard of Gordon (1285-1318) and Gentile da Foligno (d. 1348).

The recently discovered fly leaf from Bruges reflects the early diffusion of the Latin text. Middle Dutch manuscript texts are an adaptation of Gilles's urine poem, including that of Johannes de Altre (also known as Jan van Aalter, fl. circa. 1350).[10] Gilles has undoubtedly contributed to the diagnostic interest in uroscopy, as would thrive in the late Middle Ages and the early modern period.

Correspondence to:
Evelien Hauwaerts: evelien.hauwaerts@brugge.be
Johan Boelaert: johan.r.boelaert@telenet.be

10

Munk J. *Een vlaemsche leringe van orinen uit de veertiende eeuw* (doktoraatsproefschrift, Leiden). A.W. Sijthoff's uitgeversmaatschappij: Leiden, 1917.

THE 100TH ANNIVERSARY OF THE JOURNAL D'UROLOGIE MÉDICALE ET CHIRURGICALE

Johan J. Mattelaer[1]

1. *Urologist in Kortrijk, Belgium, Member of the History Office of the EAU*

In 1882, the first issue of 'Annales des maladies des organes génito-urinaires' was published. In 1912, exactly 100 years ago, the 'Annales' were replaced by the 'Journal d'Urologie médicale et chirurgicale with Marion and Heitz Boyer as editors-in-chief.

We analysed the complete volume I (January – June 1912). Interesting is that the first article, written by Pousson, gives a complete overview of stone disease through history. In the following number (15 February 1912) we can read a very impressive obituary of Prof. Albarran, who passed away in January 1912 and starts with the words: Vous êtes de ceux qui sont destinés à vivre après leur mort.[You are one who is destined to live on after death.]

In a study of the whole first volume of the Journal, we are able to give an excellent overview of the evolution in urology and the high scientific standards a century ago. One of the items is an interesting paper 'le radiodiagnostic en urologie' par G. Maingot.

JOURNAL D'UROLOGIE
MÉDICALE ET CHIRURGICALE

Publié tous les mois par MM.

F. GUYON

CARLIER — LEGUEU — POUSSON — F. WIDAL
(Lille) (Paris) (Bordeaux) (Paris)

DESNOS — JEANBRAU — MICHON — RAFIN
(Paris) (Montpellier) (Paris) (Lyon)

RÉDACTEURS EN CHEF, MM.

MARION (Paris) — HEITZ-BOYER (Paris)

SECRÉTAIRE DE LA RÉDACTION

SAINT-CÈNE

Tome I — Janvier-Juin 1912

MASSON ET CIE, ÉDITEURS
LIBRAIRES DE L'ACADÉMIE DE MÉDECINE
120, BOULEVARD SAINT-GERMAIN, PARIS

TABLE ALPHABÉTIQUE DES MATIÈRES

PAR NOMS D'AUTEURS

CONTENUES DANS LE TOME I [1]

Bazy (P.). — La pyélotomie dans les calculs du rein [M. O.] 739
Boeckel (A.). — De l'exclusion de la vessie dans la tuberculose réno-vésicale [M O.] 345
Botez (Georges). — Considérations sur la pathologie et la chirurgie du rein en fer à cheval [M. O.]. 193, 373, 503, 633
Bourcy (P.) et Legueu (F.). — Un grand kyste de la capsule surrénale [M. O.]. 181
Constantinesco (G.). — L'incontinence d'urine symptomatique de la tuberculose rénale [M. O.]. 611
Desnos (E.). — Corps étranger d'origine appendiculaire simulant un calcul vésical [R. F.]. 517
Gayet (G.). — Résection orthopédique du bassinet pour hydronéphrose à crises intermittentes. Résultat après deux ans [R. F.]. 625
Grégoire (Raymond). — Hydronéphrose dans un rein en fer à cheval. Urétéropexie. Guérison [R. F.] ...
Heitz-Boyer (M.). — Diagnostic rapide de la tuberculose urinaire par une nouvelle méthode : réation de l'antigène dans les urines (Debré et Paraf) [T. U.] 71
— (J.). — J. Albarran (1860-1912) [M. O.]. 165
— et Hovelacque (A.). — Création d'une nouvelle vessie et d'un nouvel urètre [T. U.]. 237
Héresco (P.) et Cealic (M.). — Le traitement des complications articulaires de la blennorragie par des injections de sérum antiméningococcique [M. O.]. 477
Hovelacque (André). — Étude anatomo-pathologique de l'exstrophie complète de la vessie [M. O.]. 43, 205
Lecène (P.) et Hovelacque (A.). — Les cancers développés sur la vessie exstrophiée [M. O.]. 493
Legueu (Félix). — Des troubles urinaires provoqués par les fibromes du col utérin [M. O.]. 33
—, Papin et Maingot. — La cystoradiographie [M. O.]. 749
Lippens (Adrien). — Guérison d'une fistule périnéo-prostatique par la pâte bismuthée [R. F.]. 781
Maingot (G.). — Le radiodiagnostic en urologie [R. G.]. 399
Marinesco (N.). — De l'épididymectomie dans la tuberculose génitale [T. U.]. 787

Marion (G.). — Evolution simultanée d'un cancer et d'une tuberculose sur le même rein [R. F.]. 67
— Un cas d'urètre double chez l'homme [R. F.] 235
— De la reconstitution de l'urètre par urétrorraphie circulaire avec dérivation de l'urine [T. U.] 523
— Sur la conduite à tenir dans les cas de tuberculose rénale où toute exploration des reins est rendue impossible par l'état de la vessie [M. O.] . 599
— Une nouvelle cause d'erreur dans la radiographie des calculs du rein [R. F.] 655
— Prostatite aiguë chez un prostatectomisé [R. F.] 783
Marsan (Félix). — Les néphrites chroniques douloureuses [R. G.]. . 85
Mériel (E.). — Volumineux prolapsus rectal dû au ténesme vésical par calcul chez un enfant [R. F.]. . . . 785
Orlowski. — L'inflammation du veru montanum et ses conséquences directes et réflexes [M. O.] 769
Périneau. — Résultats actuels du traitement des urétéro-pyélonéphrites suppurées par le cathétérisme urétéral et les lavages du bassinet [R. G.]. 664
Pousson. — L'affection calculeuse à travers les âges [M. O.] 1
Rafin. — L'asepsie et l'infection des urines tuberculeuses [M. O.] 777
— Mode de début de la tuberculose rénale [M. O.]. 779
Rendu (Robert). — Dilatation kystique intra-vésicale de l'extrémité inférieure de l'uretère : hydronéphrose congénitale par sténose des méats urétéraux [R. F.]. 393
Rochet. — La dérivation urinaire temporaire (par l'hypogastre et le périnée) dans les opérations sur l'urètre [M. O.]. 593
Vignard (P.) et Thévenot (Léon). — La tuberculose rénale chez l'enfant [M. O.] 323
Widal (F.), Lemierre (A.) et Ambard (A.). — Études des échanges urinaires et particulièrement de l'excrétion uréique dans un cas d'albuminurie orthostatique [M. O.]. 27
— et Weill (A.). — La péricardite des brightiques, ses rapports avec l'azotémie [M. O.]. 177
— et Bénard (R.). — Pyélonéphrite gravidique descendante par septicémie coli-bacillaire [M. O.] 313

---

[1]. Cette table mentionne l'indication des Mémoires originaux (M. O.), les Recueils de faits (R. F.), les Techniques urinaires (T. U.), les Revues générales (R. G.).

JOURNAL D'UROLOGIE. — I.   58

JOURNAL D'UROLOGIE

MÉMOIRES ORIGINAUX

L'AFFECTION CALCULEUSE A TRAVERS LES AGES

Par le Professeur **POUSSON**.

(*Leçon d'ouverture de l'année scolaire 1911-1912.*)

L'étude des affections des voies urinaires, plus que celle des maladies des autres organes et appareils de l'économie, a bénéficié des progrès prestigieux réalisés dans les diverses branches des sciences au cours des vingt-cinq dernières années du xixe siècle, progrès qui, depuis que nous sommes entrés dans le xxe, s'exaltent encore par le concours que se prêtent les multiples découvertes du génie humain. C'est qu'en effet, l'urologie, puisque cette dénomination est définitivement et justement acquise désormais en nosologie, non seulement exige, pour être cultivée avec fruit, les connaissances de l'anatomie et de la physiologie normales et pathologiques si complexes de l'appareil urinaire et les notions approfondies de l'histologie, de la cytologie, de la microbiologie, mais elle est, en outre, largement tributaire de la chimie et de la physique. L'application à l'uropathologie des conquêtes de ces deux dernières sciences, auxquelles on ne saurait, sans injustice, conserver plus longtemps l'épithète d'accessoires, a jeté un jour nouveau sur bien des troubles naguère inconnus dans leur essence et partant sans thérapeutique précise et efficace. Grâce aux procédés de plus en plus perfectionnés de l'analyse, qui permet de déceler dans les urines les variations de ses éléments normaux et

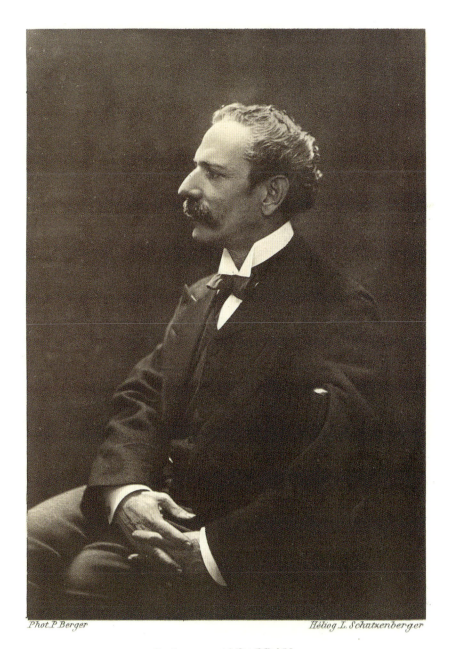

Professeur ALBARRAN
(1860 - 1912)

J. ALBARRAN

— 1860-1912 —

« Vous êtes de ceux qui sont destinés à vivre après leur mort. » Ces émouvantes paroles, qu'en un douloureux adieu le professeur Guyon adressait à son élève bien-aimé, comme elles traduisaient l'impression de tous devant la tombe ouverte du Maître qui vient de disparaître, expriment le sentiment que j'éprouve en commençant cette étude.

Dans le cimetière de Neuilly, où nous lui rendions un suprême hommage d'affectueuse admiration, de touchants discours ont dit sa lumineuse intelligence, sa débordante activité, sa volonté indomptable, sa droiture, son grand cœur, toutes les nobles qualités qui faisaient d'Albarran un être d'élite, un de ces hommes qui inspirent à ceux qui les approchent un culte fervent et durable.

Il appartient à ce Journal, où il fit paraître tant de beaux travaux, de rappeler le développement magnifique de sa vie scientifique, de montrer quelle œuvre de vérité, et par cela impérissable, ce Maître a su bâtir en un temps trop court. On pardonnera à une tendre affection d'évoquer parfois des détails de la vie intime : ce sera pour mieux faire comprendre la formation et l'évolution de cette nature exceptionnelle.

*
* *

On sait sa naissance à Cuba, dans une petite ville de la partie occidentale de l'île, Sagua-la-Grande. Orphelin de bonne heure, ses premiers guides intellectuels furent son parrain, ancien chirurgien espagnol, qui le protégea pendant toute son enfance, et un frère aîné, médecin aussi, Pedro Albarran, esprit remarquablement fin et distingué. Elevé, pendant quelque temps, dans un collège de la Havane, il arrivait en Espagne à l'âge de neuf ans. A treize ans, il était reçu bachelier, à dix-sept ans, licencié en médecine, à dix-neuf ans, docteur de la Faculté de Madrid avec la mention « hors de pair ». Pourvu du diplôme, il n'avait pas

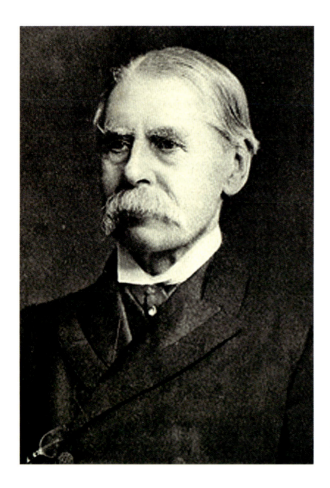

Figure 1:
Sir Henry Thompson,
Bt. (1820 - 1904).

OPEN CYSTOTOMY FOR BLADDER CANCER. FROM NECESSITY TO OBSCURITY; THE RISE AND FALL OF A HISTORICAL OPERATION.

Susannah M. La-Touche [1], Roger C. Kockelbergh [2] Jonathan C. Goddard [3]

1. BSc MBBS MRCS, Urology Registrar, Department of Urology, Leicester General Hospital.

2. DM FRCS(Ed) FRCS(Urol), Consultant Urological Surgeon, Department of Urology, Leicester General Hospital

3. MD FRCS (Eng) FRCS (Urol) FEBU, Consultant Urological Surgeon, Department of Urology, Leicester General Hospital

[1] Thompson, H. "On a case of Tumour of the Bladder (in the male) successfully removed through a perineal section of the urethra." *Medico-Churgical Transactions*. 1882; 65:147-53.

[2] Freyer, P.J. *Clinical Lectures on the Surgical Diseases of the Urinary Organs*. New York: Wood; 1908.

[3] Milner, W.A. "The role of conservative surgery in the treatment of bladder tumours." *British Journal of Urology*. 1954;26(4):375-84.

Introduction

In 1882, Sir Henry Thompson stated that opening the bladder to remove tumours was a lifesaving procedure.[1] Sir Peter Freyer claimed it was the only way to prevent the bleeding, pain and suffering of these patients.[2] So, the open treatment of bladder tumours by suprapubic cystotomy was born of necessity. However, by 1954, William Milner described this procedure as an outdated operation[3] and now we would be horrified by the concept of purposely opening a bladder containing a transitional cell tumour.

We examine the appearance, rise and decline of open cystotomy for the treatment of bladder cancer. Primary and secondary sources were examined from the 1880s until the 1980s, documenting the history of this procedure.

The need for open treatment of bladder cancer

In the nineteenth century, patients with superficial bladder cancer lived a miserable existence. They suffered from recurrent intractable haematuria and painful frequent micturition. Sir Henry Thompson, the famous Victorian urologist (Fig.1) suggested bladder instillations of the astringent silver nitrate for the bleeding. As for the pain he writes in some desperation:

"…do not spare opiates—trying any form, or all forms in turn, until you find that which most assuages it …It is not a question of saving life, but a question of mitigating that most frightful of human miseries prolonged, continuous, severe bodily suffering; and this for a patient whose doom is certain, and to whom life has come to be for the most part a dire calamity."[4]

Establishing the diagnosis of bladder tumours was difficult. Haematuria, the most common symptom, often led to a suspicion of bladder stone. The interior of the bladder was explored blindly with a metal sound but, unlike the hard stone, the soft yielding bladder tumour was difficult to detect. Occasionally bladder tumours were discovered incidentally at perineal lithotomy procedures.

This was the case on 6 November 1880, when Sir Henry Thompson carried out a median perineal lithotomy on 29 year-old Thomas Reading. He was surprised to find a "chestnut-sized" tumour on the fundus, which he twisted off with forceps.[1] Thompson noted that others before him, such as Professor Murray Humphry in 1879[5] and Davies-Collins in 1880,[6] had also carried out this procedure and he fully advocated it as a treatment.

Thompson also quoted the case of the Prussian surgeon Theodor Billroth who had removed a large tumour from the bladder by the suprapubic route. The patient was a boy of 12, with frequent painful micturition. A tumour could be palpated in the region of the bladder.

4
Thompson, H. *Diseases of the Urinary Organs. Second ed.* London: Churchill; 1869.

5
Humphry, G.M. "Tumour in the Bladder removed by Perineal Incision; complete recovery." *Medico-Churgical Transactions.* 1879;62:421-7.

6
Davies-Colley, J.N.C. "Villous growth of the bladder successfully removed by perineal incision." Transactions of the Clinical Society of London. 1880;14:104.

A lateral perineal incision into the bladder was made, and a tumour, nearly of the size of a fist (a myo-sarcoma) was found.

Owing to its size it was found impossible to extract through the perineum so a suprapubic incision was made, both recti were cut across, and a transverse incision carried into the bladder. The tumour was then torn through, near its base, with the finger, and the pedicle dissected out. In a month the patient was discharged perfectly well.[5]

The Suprapubic approach

Historically, abdominal wounds led to significant morbidity and, more often than not, mortality. The bladder was considered part of this rule, probably because of the failure to distinguish its extraperitoneal nature when full. Suprapubic incisions would often result in urinary contamination and peritonitis. An incision into the peritoneum of a straining struggling unanaesthetised patient could lead to an extrusion of irreplaceable bowel.

Pierre Franco (1505-1578) has been credited with the earliest case report of deliberate suprapubic surgery successfully removing a stone this way at Lausanne in 1561.[7] James Douglas, very accurately described the approaches to the bladder before the Royal Society of London in 1718 and his brother John Douglas used this knowledge to remove four stones suprapubically between December 1719 and March 1721 at the Westminster Hospital.

His three out of four success rate gained him the FRS and freedom of the Barbers

[7] Parrott, J. "Suprapubic Cystotomy vs. Perineal Section." *JAMA*. 1899;32(7):356-9.

Company, the City of London and a job at the Westminster. John taught William Cheselden who began using this method from 1722 and in 1723 he published his Treatise on the High Operation for the Stone. But Cheselden soon changed from this approach back to the perineal approach. This may have been because of the new challenge presented by this novel approach, or because of the significant morbidity associated with the suprapubic route. Certainly, the technique was slow to become established.

By 1886 however, Sir Henry Thompson wrote "The high operation for opening the bladder has in my opinion, been rendered so safe and efficient by certain modifications recently made as to deserve the careful attention of all practical surgeons".[8] By this time, he had used it to remove two bladder tumours.

[8] Thompson, H. *On the suprapubic operation of opening the bladder for the stone and for tumours*. London: Churchill; 1886.

Sir Peter Freyer (1851 - 1921) of St Peter's Hospital in London, adopted the suprapubic approach because of better visualisation.[2] These techniques cured or palliated the suffering of patients previously inadequately treated with astringents and washouts.

The technique of open cystotomy

Patients were positioned in either supine or Trendelenburg's position. The bladder was often distended with a small volume of water and the rectum with an inflatable elastic air-bag (Peterson's bag). The aim in doing so was to make the bladder more prominent and to increase the suprapubic space. By 1895, this practice of rectal distension had largely been abandoned, having caused rupture of the bladder and bowel on many occasions, usually discovered at post mortem examination. With Trendelenburg's position there were some advantages, as the intestinal pressure tended to gravitate toward the thorax and away from the wound.

The surgeon would open the bladder, using either a vertical or transverse incision. The vertical incision beginning immediately above the pubis continued for two inches toward the umbilicus in the midline. This was carried down to the intermuscular interval, which was opened and an index finger was used to draw the peritoneal reflection toward the umbilicus. Using this technique, the peritoneum was seldom visualised. Fat and cellular tissue between the muscle and the bladder was 'scraped away with the finger', until the anterior surface of the bladder was seen. It was advisable to either avoid or tie any large veins and to use a stay-suture through the bladder wall to secure it.

The scalpel would then be inserted into the bladder in the midline, and the incision made in an upward direction to allow insertion of the index finger. If the stay sutures were not grasped and water allowed to escape the bladder would become floppy and, in these cases, it was recommended that a metal bulbous-ended bougie should be passed into the bladder, when the opening is found.[7]

A transverse incision could also be made immediately above, and parallel with, the line of the pubis. Trendelenburg recommended that the mucous membrane of the bladder should be connected with the skin by means of temporary sutures. This incision was recommended in some cases of tubercular ulceration of the bladder requiring local treatment and for removing extensive growths. However, many believed

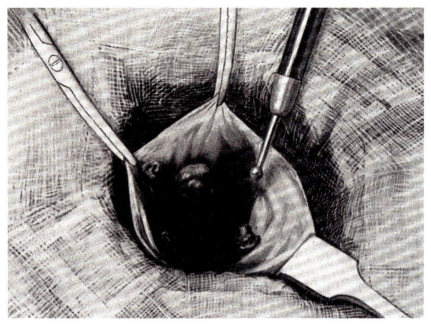

Figure 2: Cystotomy allowing the visualisation of bladder tumours prior to treatment by cautery (from Beer, E., Tumours of the urinary bladder. London: Baillière, Tindall & Cox; 1935.

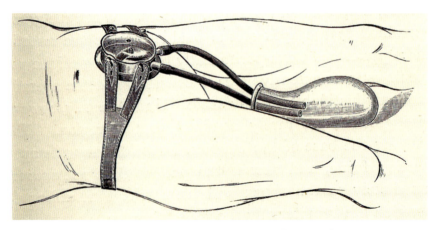

Figure 3: The Hamilton Irving Box for draining suprapubic wounds (from Freyer PJ. Clinical Lectures on the Surgical Diseases of the Urinary Organs. New York: Wood; 1908.)

that the transverse incision was more likely to result in a ventral hernia.

Bladder tumours were palpated by finger and could also be inspected by opaque glass or vulcanite specula of different sizes introduced through the wound, as described by Hurry Fenwick in conjunction with the 'reflection from the electric light'. Watson's spring wire speculum was also used to keep the bladder open and some scoops and an elm cleator hook were often kept to hand. Using this combination of techniques and instruments bladder tumours could be removed with a greater degree of precision. (Fig. 2) Freyer used an electric headlamp to improve vision.[2]

For haemostasis, iron, turpentine, or the wires of a galvanic cautery were used, or hot water and hazeline injected through the wound for more minor bleeding.

At this time the issue of wound closure following suprapubic cystotomy was contentious. In some cases, suturing the bladder wall and superficial wound resulted in primary wound closure, but it would often lead to infection, inflammation and urine leak.

Stedman 1985 described leaving the bladder opening alone and closing the superficial wound to some extent, to allow space for a 'Guyon's double drainage-tube'. This was comprised of two rubber catheters connected together, which give access either way either to antiseptic lotion or urine, the latter being received in a bottle by the patient's side.[9] Freyer used a large bore suprapubic drainage tube, but also described the unusual looking Hamilton Irving Box.[2] (Fig. 3)

9
Stedman, T. *Twentieth Century Practice: Diseases of the uropoietic system. Vol 1*. California: Wood; 1895.

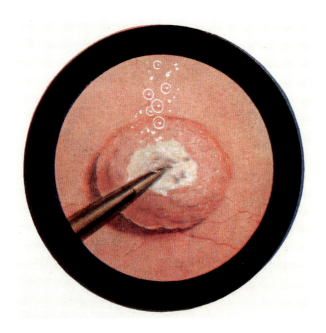

Figure 4: Cystoscopic fulguration of a bladder tumour (from Canny Ryall, E, Operative Cystoscopy, London: Klinpton; 1925).

The invention of the cystoscope

In 1879, Max Nitze developed the first usable cystoscope. This allowed easier diagnosis of bladder tumours. Their fimbriae were seen to wave in the current of the irrigating fluid of Freyer's cystoscope "presenting a bright pink appearance of rare beauty".[2]

The new cystoscopes were used promptly for treatment as well as diagnosis and soon, both snares and forceps were designed for endoscopic use on bladder tumours. By 1908, Casper was only advocating suprapubic tumour removal for those that could not be treated conservatively (that is, palliatively) or the lesion could not be removed via the female urethra with forceps or cystoscopically.

In 1910, Edwin Beer of America published his fulguration technique for bladder tumours using the Oudin current.[10] (Fig. 4) On his return from Vienna to New York, after he observed Nitze's work, he conducted his own research. The Wappler Brothers made for him the necessary instruments.[11]

In 1915, Kretschmer stated that fulguration of bladder tumours (after Beer 1910) had displaced all other methods.[12] It is possible, as with the advent of so many new technologies in urological history, that the excitement of the new technology prevailed, leading to somewhat premature conclusions.

The cystoscope and subsequent Sterne-McCarthy resectoscope should have ended open cystotomy, and indeed its golden age was from the 1880's until the 1930's, but the technique continued.

According to Hurry Fenwick, the incandescent lamp cystoscope of Nitze or Leiter is an instrument of real practical utility, by means of which the whole cavity may be visually inspected. However, in 1888, he declared that the cystoscope had not yet attracted its due attention in England and, to that end, published an article outlining the cystoscope of that time as 'simpler, safer and more successful than its progenitors of 1862 and 1879-80.'[13]

The reluctance to adopt the cystoscope may have been due to the problems and expense

10
Beer, E. "Removal of neoplasms of the urinary bladder." *JAMA.* 1910;54(22):1768-9.

11
Wade, H. "Urological Reflections". *Proc R Soc Med.* 1946; 39(11):751-4.

12
Kretschmer, H. "Fulguration treatment of tumors of the bladder." *JAMA.* 1915; 64(13):1050-2.

13
Fenwick, E.H. "The Electric Illumination of the Male Bladder by Means of the New Incandescent-Lamp Cystoscope." *British Medical Journal.* 1888;1(1414):240-1.

encountered with previous models compared to the speed and anatomical simplicity of a well-known open operation. In addition, personal experiences of these instruments was limited and many advised extensive practice on cadavers and artificial bladders, before attempting the procedure on patients.[14]

14
Smith, J. *Abdominal Surgery*. 25th ed. London: Churchill; 1896.

Transition from open cystotomy to TURBT

In the 1890s there were two schools of thought for the treatment of these tumours. The USA favoured perineal and urethral surgery and Europe favoured the suprapubic route. By 1893 Fenwick published a paper demonstrating that surgeons would use cystoscopy for diagnosis, but would resort to the familiar suprapubic (or in some cases perineal) incision for treatment of bladder tumours.[15]

15
Fenwick, E.H. "Clinical Lecture on One Hundred Cases of Tumours of the Urinary Bladder: Delivered at the London Hospital." *British Medical Journal*. 1893;1(1693):1209-12.

Towards the early to mid-20th century, there seemed to be more of a realisation of the full benefits of cystoscopy, and so the evolution to what we know as the modern TURBT really began. By 1950, fewer open suprapubic procedures and more cystoscopy with diathermy or fulgaration were being performed. The suprapubic route was often reserved for when accessibility was an issue and a cystoscope could not be passed.[16]

16
Band, D. "Vesical tumours An analysis of a personal series". *BJUI*. 1950; 22 (4): 381-393

There was a comprehension that endoscopy could offer early diagnosis, rather than clearance via suprapubic cystotomy as a response to an overtly palpable bladder mass. Cystoscopy also offered good clearance of the tumour base, inspection of the rest of the bladder and benefits in palliation. Indeed by 1954 suprapubic cystotomy and fulgaration had an operative mortality of 25%, which was unjustifiable compared to that of TUR at 0.3%.[3]

However, evolution of histological classification meant that the more common newly-defined papillary growths were the only tumours that could be treated by early endoscopists with any degree of success.[17] So, despite claims by Milner that open cystotomy was an outdated procedure, it continued for a few years more.

In Britain, even during the second half of the twentieth century, many urological procedures were carried out by general surgeons with an interest in urology, rather than by specialist urologists. Perhaps this led to an inclination to reach for a scalpel rather than a cystoscope.

Using the open approach to place radioactive seeds

The operation of cystotomy for bladder tumours was subsequently combined with the insertion of radioactive seeds into the tumour base. This may have been another reason that the open technique lingered. The practice was begun in the early twentieth century. Schüller claimed that he was the first to use radon in Vienna in 1913. However, the first published cases were to be found in the first volume of the Journal of Urology in 1917, by Young in collaboration with Frontz.[18] The conclusion was that it was only suitable for malignant tumours failing to respond to fulguration.

The first instrument for radon seed implantation was constructed by Neill in 1922, but prior to 1939 this form of treatment was not really considered to be important for treating bladder cancer. Hutchinson in 1935 published a guide to proper dosage and implantation, borne from the realization that the diminishing popularity of this treatment modality was principally due to incorrect dosage.

---

17 Herr, H.W. "Early history of endoscopic treatment of bladder tumours from Grunfeld's Polypenkneipe to the Stern-McCarthy resectoscope". *Journal of Endourology.* 2006; 20(2): 85-91.

18 Young, H.H. and W.A. Frontz. "Some new methods in the treatment of carcinoma of the lower genitourinary tract with radium." *The Journal of Urology.* 1917;1:505-41.

From 1968 radon seeds were not readily available, so the transition to radioactive gold grains was made.[19] Radio-gold grains 198Au (half-life 2.69 days) were permanently implanted by a gold grain gun, while hairpin-bent radiotantalum wires 182 (half-life 111 days) were temporarily introduced by a special instrument with the bent end of the wires facing the urethra and with a string attached to this bent end to facilitate easy removal through the urethra.[20] This practice continued until at least the 1970s.[21]

The improvements in Cystectomy survival, the Hopkins lens and the end of open cystotomy for TCC

Early cystectomies were associated with a high operative mortality. In 1923 Scheele reported 60 operations from the literature with operative mortality up to 53.5%, but by the 1960s this had been reduced to 10-15%.[22] Reports of operative mortality as low as 5.4%, significant for that time, were published in 1963 from a series of 146 operations. Despite these improvements cystectomy was performed with some degree of hesitancy in the 1970s and recommended only as a salvage procedure after initial treatment had failed.[22]

In 1967, Karl Stortz, the German instrument maker, produced the first commercially available cystoscope using the Hopkins rod lens system. The rod lens, designed by British Professor Harold Hopkins, gave better light transmission resulting in brighter images with better contrast and colour.[23] This led to a much improved ability to fulgurate and resect tumours transurethrally.

19
Dix, V.W., W. Shanks, G.C. Tressider, J.P. Blandy, HF Hope-Stone HFand B.G.F. Shepheard. "Carcinoma of the Bladder; Treatment by diathermy snare excision and interstitial radiation." *British Journal of Urology.* 1970;42:213-28.

20
Fitchart, T. and A.G. Sandison. "Management of urinary bladder cancer." *South African Medical Journal.* 1978;54(18):731-40.

21
Bullock, N. Personal Communication. 2012. Ref Type: Personal Communication

22
Poole-Wilson, D.S., and R.J. Barnard. "Total Cystectomy for bladder tumours." *British Journal of Urology.* 1971;43:16-24.

23
Cockett, W.S. and A.T.K. Cockett. "The Hopkins Rod-lens system and the Stortz cold light illumination system." *Urology.* 1998;51(Supp 5A):1-2.

The introduction of the Hopkins rod lens system and subsequent modifications with the Stern-McCarthy resectoscope, combined with improvements in the mortality of cystectomy for invasive disease meant open cystotomy for treatment of bladder tumours gradually became a historical operation.

Conclusion

The modern urologist would avoid opening a bladder containing tumour. In the nineteenth century open cystotomy to remove bladder tumours was a pioneering innovation. The risks of opening the abdomen or of tumour seeding were accepted in an attempt to alleviate the suffering of these unfortunate patients. What seems more surprising is perhaps the longevity of this practice.

Despite the invention of the cystoscope and the introduction of endoscopic fulgaration and resection of bladder tumours, the open technique continued until the 1970's, particularly in Britain and Europe. The death knell of the open technique was sounded by the introduction of the Hopkins rod lens with its superior visualisation. The practice of open cystotomy to remove bladder tumours lasted for about a century and is now forgotten chapter in the history of urology.

Correspondence to:
Dr. Jonathan C. Goddard
Department of Urology
Leicester General Hospital
Gwendolen Road, Leicester, LE5 4PW
United Kingdom
+44(0)1162584448
jonathan.goddard@uhl-tr.nhs.uk

UROLOGY IN FRANCE IN THE 19TH CENTURY AND THE BEGINNING OF THE 20TH CENTURY

An overview of the birth of urology

Philip E.V. Van Kerrebroeck[1]

1. *Urologist in Maastricht, the Netherlands, Member of the History Office of the EAU*

During the 19th century and the beginning of the 20th century, France played an important role in the development of urology as a separate clinical and scientific specialty. Starting with surgeons who were further developing uro-genital surgery, through the creation of a specific ward for "urological" patients to the establishment of a new sub-specialty, entitled "urology", but still within the field of surgery: all of this happened in France over the course of the 19th century.

Hence it is worthwhile to review where these intriguing events found their origin and how they can be situated in the framework of a country going through major changes at all levels of society. However, these developments are also the work of individual men that devoted their life to the establishment of what we now call "our specialty".

France in the 19th Century and early 20th Century

France went through many changes over the course of the 19th century and as a consequence developed only slowly from a rural to a more industrialised society. Politically, the 19th century was a period of many changes and revolutions that significantly influenced the lives of individuals. These events also had an important

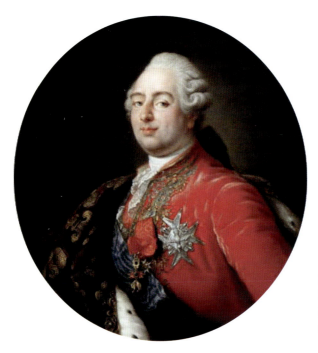

Figure 1:
Louis XVI de France
(Antoine-François
Callet, 1786).

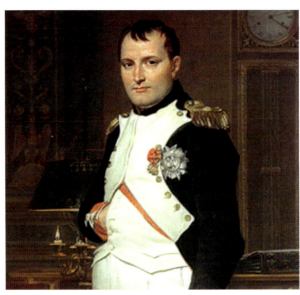

Figure 2:
Napoleon Bonaparte
(Jacques Louis David,
1912).

influence on the work and working conditions of physicians of that time.

In order to understand the importance of some of the medical developments during the 19th century, and in order to imagine the daily life situation of our colleagues of that time, before discussing the developments of urology in France in the 19th century, we will present an overview on the politics, the geography, the demographics and the cultural life in France during the 19th century.

Politics

The 19th century starts in France with the Revolution of 1789 and ends with the outbreak of World War I in 1914.[1] Events in-between include the First Republic (1792-1799), the First Empire (1804-1814), the Restoration (1814-1830), the July Monarchy (1830-1848), the Second Republic (1848-1852), the Second Empire (1852-1870) and partly the Third Republic (1870-1914-1940).

The First French Republic was proclaimed in 1792 after the Revolution, and lasted till 1799. In 1793, King Louis XVI (1754-1793) (Fig. 1) was condemned to death and executed. His wife Marie Antoinette was also beheaded later that year. Under the new constitution, Bicameral legislature was established and soon Napoleon Bonaparte (1769-1821) (Fig. 2) installed the Consulate in the "coup d'état" of 1799. Three years later, Napoleon became the First Consul and dictator for life. The Senate proclaimed him Emperor in 1804. This was the start of the First French Empire that existed from 1804 till 1814.

---

[1] Wright, G. *France in Modern Times*, New York, 1987.

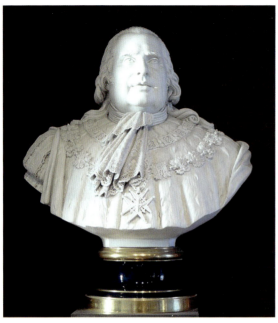

Figure 3: Louis XVIII of France (Jean Brachard, 1823).

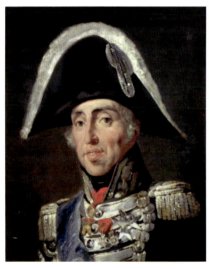

Figure 4: Charles X, king of France and Navarre (Horace Vernet, 1826).

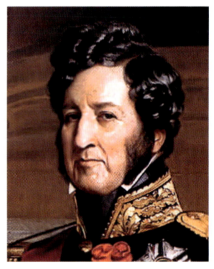

Figure 5: King Louis-Philippe of France (Franz Winterhalter, 1841).

During this period, France was a global power, reorganising territorial boundaries in continental Europe and territories outside France. The only country in Europe that didn't bow down before the French dictator was Great Britain. Napoleon attempted to defeat the British Navy during the Battle of Trafalgar in 1805, but he failed. He resorted to economic warfare strategies, establishing an embargo on trade with Britain soon thereafter.

The effect of this embargo turned out to be much worse for Napoleon's allies than for Britain. Russia suffered particularly. Russia resumed trade with Britain in 1812, which resulted in Napoleon's invasion of Russia. This campaign was disastrous for the French. Ultimately it led to Napoleon's abdication in 1814. He was exiled and sent to the island of Elba. In 1815, he briefly returned to power, but after he lost the Battle of Waterloo, he was exiled permanently to the island of St Helena, where he died.

Following these events, the Bourbon Dynasty returned to power. This period is known as the French Restoration (1814-1830). The governing monarchs, starting with Louis XVIII (1755-1824) (Fig. 3) came to rule over a greatly transformed France. His successor, Charles X (1757-1836) (Fig. 4) instigated very conservative policies, which caused civil unrest, culminating in the July Revolution of 1830. As a result, the king fled the country and was replaced by Louis-Philippe d'Orleans (1773-1850) (Fig. 5).

His reign was known as the July Monarchy (1830-1848). At this time, the bourgeoisie was dominant, and France enjoyed a flourishing

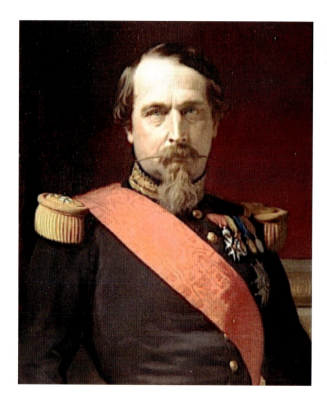

Figure 6: Napoleon III (Franz Winterhalter, 1855).

economy. However it also experienced social turmoil. The monarchy fell with the Revolution of 1848, and the Second Republic (1848-1852) was proclaimed that year. Charles Louis Napoleon Bonaparte (1808-1873), a nephew of Napoleon I, was elected president in 1848. Three years later he staged a coup, and in 1852 was declared Emperor Napoleon III. (Fig. 6)

Thus started the Second Empire (1852-1870), which lasted until 1870. It was an epoch of great urbanisation, industrialisation and economic growth. However, Napoleon III's foreign policymaking was problematic, partly due to his health problems related to bladder stones and subsequent uraemia. (Fig. 7) (See also: Van Kerrebroeck, "Auguste Nelaton" in *De Historia* vol 19.) Conflicts with Prussia provoked the Franco-Prussian War of 1870. Eventually, France capitulated and Napoleon III was captured.

This led to the creation of the Third French Republic (1870–1940). It would go on to last longer than all other French governments since the Revolution. The revolt of the Paris Commune (1871) was suppressed violently during the tenure of the Royalists (1871-1879) and hundreds of republican rebels were killed in the Père Lachaise cemetery during the so-called "Bloody Week". In 1879, the Opportunists (1879-1899) succeeded the Royalists till the Radicals (1899-1914) took power in 1899. During their tenure, France acquired many overseas territories and implemented many domestic reforms, especially in the field of education. A modern, 20th century nation-state was forged.

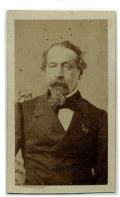

Figure 7:
The ill Napoleon III
(Georges Spingler, 1860-1865).

Geography

At the time of the French Revolution (1789), France had expanded to nearly her modern territorial limits. The 19th century would complete the process with the annexation of the Duchy of Savoy and the city of Nice and some small papal and foreign possessions. In 1830, France invaded Algeria, and in 1848 this North African country was fully integrated into France as a "département". The late 19th century saw France embark on a massive programme of overseas imperialism, including French Indochina (modern day Cambodia, Vietnam and Laos) and Africa (most of North-West and Central Africa). With the French defeat in the Franco-Prussian War of 1870, France however lost the provinces of Alsace and portions of Lorraine to Germany and these would only be regained at the end of World War I.²

2

Weber, E. *Peasants into Frenchmen: the modernisation of rural France.* London, 1979.

Demographics

Between 1795 and 1866, metropolitan France was the 2nd most populous country of Europe, behind Russia and between 1866 and 1911, France was the 3rd one, behind Russia and Germany. Unlike other European countries, France did not experience a strong population growth from the middle of the 19th century to the first half of the 20th century. Until 1850, population growth was mainly in the countryside, but a period of massive urbanisation began under the Second Empire. (Fig. 8) Industrialization was a late phenomenon in France because the Napoleonic wars had hindered early industrialisation.

Hence France's economy in the 1830s had not developed sufficiently to support industrial expansion. By the revolution of 1848, a growing industrial workforce began to participate actively in French politics, but their hopes were largely betrayed by the policies of the Second Empire. The loss of the important coal, steel and glass production regions of Alsace and Lorraine would cause further problems. France remained a rather rural country in the early 1900s. (Fig. 9)

France's rate of urbanisation was still well behind other European countries. However in the 19th century, France was a country of immigration for political refugees from Eastern Europe (Germany, Poland, Hungary,

Russia, and Ashkenazi Jews) and from the Mediterranean (Italy, Spanish Sephardic Jews and North-African Mizrahi Jews). France was the first country in Europe to emancipate its Jewish population and by 1872, there were an estimated 86,000 Jews living in the country.[2]

Language, Identity and Culture

Linguistically, France was a patchwork. People in the countryside spoke various dialects and France would only become a linguistically unified country by the end of the 19th century. From an illiteracy rate of 33% among peasants in 1870, by 1914 almost all French could read and understand the national language, although 50% still understood or spoke a regional language. Through the educational, social and military policies of the Third Republic, by 1914 the French had been converted from a "country of peasants into a nation of Frenchmen". By 1914, most French could read French and the use of regional languages had greatly decreased. The role of the Catholic Church in public life had been radically altered and a sense of national identity and pride was actively taught.[3]

The 19th century was to be a turning point for French art, and for art around the world, especially during the latter part of the century.[4] From the emergence of Delacroix in the early 19th century to the surrealists 100 years later, France was to dominate the art scene. The established art school in France at the beginning of the 19th century was represented by Jacques-Louis David and Jean Ingres (Fig. 10) and had two main characteristics, great attention to fine detail and focus on painting 'proper' subjects, such as portraits of the great and good and ruined buildings in idyllic settings.

---

[3] Robb, G. *The Discovery of France: A Historical Geography, from the Revolution to the First World War*. New York, Norton, 2007.

[4] Wylie, L. and J-F. Brière, *Les Français*. 3rd edition. Prentice Hall, 2001.

The focus of the art world in the middle of the 19th century was in questioning whether this was the correct approach to painting. Ferdinand Delacroix and Theodore Gericault, leaders of the romantic art movement in France, were among the first to question the priorities of the art being painted at that time, and adopted a style that was more interested in catching the spirit of the subject rather than every fine detail. The second characteristic, what should or should not be painted, was challenged by Jean Francois Millet, who painted peasants working in the fields rather than nobles sat by a window.

These trends continued with Gustave Courbet, who was adamant that he would paint what he wanted, in the way he wanted. The next stage in the development of art was to fall to one of Courbet's 'disciples', Edouard Manet, and his colleagues. The second half of the 19th century saw the birth of impressionism rejecting once and for all a belaboured style, for fragile transitive effects of light as captured outdoors in changing light. Major representatives of this movement are Claude Monet with his cathedrals and haystacks (Fig. 11), Pierre-Auguste Renoir with both his early outdoor festivals and his later feathery style of ruddy nudes, and Edgar Degas with his dancers and bathers. They prepared the changes in visual arts during the early 20th century.

The history of 19th century French literature is that of a country struggling to deal with the aftermath of the 1789 revolution. Two republics, several revolutions and coups d'état, the empires of Napoleon I and Napoleon III, and the restoration of the monarchy followed one another in a topsy-turvy succession of regimes, ideologies, and political philosophies.

Similarly, the literary history of the 19th century is of a series of efforts to replace the classicism of the 18th century and its emphasis on order, reason, and clarity. Romanticism, realism, naturalism, Parnassianism, and symbolism were the concepts, movements, and schools that dominated. The novel continued to prosper and provided some of the masterpieces of French literature. It was the preeminent democratic genre, documenting detail and fact rather than the universal and general principles that the 18th century philosophers pursued. Liberated from the hierarchy of the old regime, the 19th century novel could express the distinctiveness of the individual. Writers increasingly portrayed protagonists from different levels of society, even the very lowest.

The turmoil of the Revolution and the Napoleonic wars did not encourage musical activity. Therefore in the early 19th century, Paris was rather a centre for musicians from other countries, such as Frederic Chopin and Franz Liszt. Music by French composers consisted mostly of inferior operas or empty, virtuosic salon pieces. A notable exception was the works of Hector Berlioz, the greatest of the French Romantics. The late 19th century saw an increase of quality in French music. Camille Saint-Saens worked for the establishment, and Cesar Franck helped restore the quality of French organ and church music. The works of Georges Bizet, Charles Gounod, and Jules Massenet brought a new spontaneity and colour to french opera. Impressionism, as seen in the music of Claude Debussy and the early works of Maurice Ravel, blossomed toward the end of the century.

The end of the 19th and the beginning of the 20th century is often termed the *belle époque*. (Fig. 12) Although associated with cultural innovations and popular amusements (cabaret, cancan, the cinema, new art forms such as Impressionism and Art Nouveau), France was nevertheless a nation divided internally on notions of religion, class, regionalisms and money, and on the international front France came repeatedly to the brink of war with the other imperial powers with all negative consequences as a result of this.

Medicine

The beginning of the 19th century in France saw its health system little changed from the middle ages. But by the end of the century, war and upheaval had altered French medicine. Revolutionary leaders condemned medical institutions and organizations, as well as doctors, but instead of the expected eradication of these institutions and professions, the movement ultimately resulted in progressive public health policies and new medical schools that produced better-educated doctors.[5]

[5] Magner, L.N. *A History of Medicine*, New York, Marcel Dekker, 1992.

The medical regulations law of 1803 stipulated a two-tier model for education. Health officers received predominantly practical training, but doctors were required to attend four years at a state medical school and pass examinations in anatomy, physiology, pathology, nosology, chemistry, pharmacy, hygiene, forensic medicine, and clinical medicine.[6] Hospital reform resulted in a milieu conducive for clinical research, autopsies, and statistical analysis. By 1830 the 30 hospitals in Paris could accommodate 20,000 patients. (Fig. 13)

[6] Bettman, O.L., *A Pictorial History of Medicine*. Springfield, Illinois, Charles C. Thomas, 1956.

In the early 19th century, a French physician might see fewer than ten patients daily, sometimes only two or three. This low utilisation of professional care was principally due to the high cost of health care compared to earnings. A visit by a health officer, who would have had less formal training than a doctor, might cost an agricultural worker a day's wage, even without a charge for the practitioner's travel. A doctor's house call could be two or three times as high. In Paris, where doctor fees were considerably more than those charged by a rural health officer, an urban artisan could pay a week's wages just for the doctor's visit.[7] Remedies cost extra, so it is not surprising that a doctor's clientele consisted mainly of landowners and their servants, merchants, other professionals, and the more successful artisans.

The practice of medicine also changed in the face of rapid advances in science, as well as new approaches by physicians. Hospital doctors began much more systematic analysis of patients' symptoms in diagnosis. Among the more powerful new techniques were anaesthesia, and the development of both antiseptic and aseptic operating theatres. Actual cures were developed for certain endemic infectious diseases. However, the decline in many of the most lethal diseases was more due to improvements in public health and nutrition than to medicine. It was not until the 20th century that the application of the scientific method to medical research began to produce multiple important developments in medicine, with great advances in pharmacology and surgery.

However medicine was revolutionised in the 19th century by advances in chemistry

---

[7] Ramsey, M. *Professional and Popular Medicine in France, 1770-1830: The Social World of Medical Practice*, Cambridge University Press, 1988.

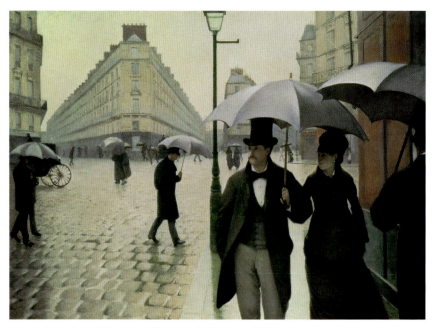

Figure 8: Paris: A Rainy Day (Gustave Caillebotte, 1877).

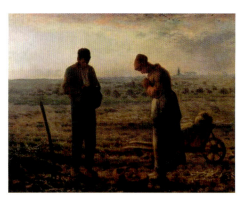

Figure 9: The Angelus, (Jean-François Millet, 1859).

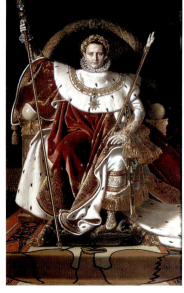

Figure 10: Napoleon on his Imperial throne, (Jean Ingres, 1806).

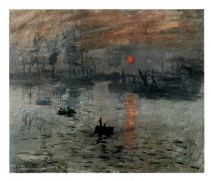

Figure 11: Impression, Soleil levant, (Claude Monet, 1873).

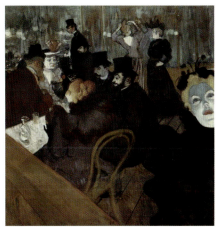

Figure 12: Au Moulin Rouge, (Henri de Toulouse-Lautrec, 1892-1895).

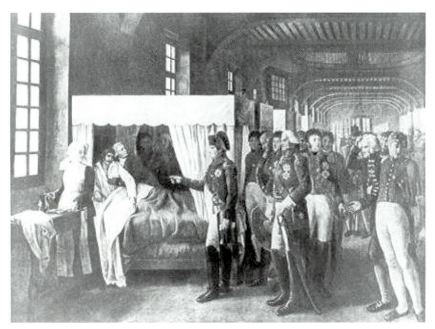

Figure 13: Napoleon visiting an hospital ward.

and laboratory techniques and equipment. Old ideas of infectious disease epidemiology were replaced with bacteriology and virology. Bacteria and microorganisms were first observed with a microscope and microbiology was initiated. The death rate of new mothers from childbed fever was significantly reduced by the simple expedient of requiring physicians to clean their hands before attending to women in childbirth.

But only since 1865 the principles of antisepsis in the treatment of wounds, a discovery by the British surgeon Joseph Lister were slowly introduced. However, medical conservatism on new breakthroughs in pre-existing science prevented them from being generally well-received during the 19th century. However, these findings were gradually supported by the discoveries made by the Frenchman Louis Pasteur (1822-1895). Linking microorganisms with disease, Pasteur brought about a revolution in medicine. He also invented, with another Frenchman Claude Bernard (1813–1878), the process of pasteurisation still in use today. His experiments confirmed the germ theory. Claude Bernard aimed at establishing the scientific method in medicine. Beside this, Pasteur founded bacteriology.

The participation of women in medical care (beyond serving as midwives, sitters and cleaning women) was very limited and only ameliorated after Florence Nightingale showed from 1852 on, in a previously male dominated profession, the elemental role of nursing in order to lessen the aggravation of patient mortality which resulted from lack of hygiene and nutrition.

We can conclude hence that during the 19th century it was not "easy" to live in France. Insecurity and anxiety governed. This general situation also influenced the individual life of the citizens and hence also the work of the medical doctors taking care of them, amongst these the urological surgeons and urologists of that time.

Urological surgery in France

Urology, which nowadays has a very definite place among the surgical specialties, had a very modest debut. We may even say that before the 18th century, the problems of the urinary tract were almost completely ignored and even opposed by the medical schools, in all countries. In ancient times and throughout the middle ages, the care of patients with "urological" problems was left in the hands of ambulant or vagabond surgeons, who performed two kinds of operation: catheterisation of urinary retention and the extraction of bladder stones.

The fact that the patients suffering from one of these two conditions were condemned to certain death, and this, in a very short time, most likely accounts for the lack of interest showed in the urinary tract by the surgeons of the first 18 centuries of our era. However even with the bad reputation of early urological surgeons, a few great names have survived the ages.

The history of urology in France is the history of urology itself because most of its realisations were brought to us by French surgeons.[8] The first important observations in urological science were made in 1250 by the French surgeon Jean Pitard (1228-1315), the first Royal Surgeon, personally serving King Louis IX, King

---
[8] Jardin, A. "The history of Urology in France". *De Historia Urologiae Europaeae*, vol 3, 11, 1996.

Philippe the Handsome and King Philippe the Brave. He performed the first serious study of the anatomy of the human kidneys, ureters and bladder, based on facts observed and described during dissections of these organs. In 1361, Guy de Chauliac (ca 1300-1368) (Fig. 14), was the first surgeon to give a clear and detailed description of the technique of perineal median cystostomy for extraction of bladder stones.

However, he was not the first surgeon to perform this operation as this was performed many centuries before his time. Ambroise Paré (ca 1510-1590), the father of surgery, completed the description of cystotomy in 1540, although his observations were only theoretical, because he never performed the operation himself. The first suprapubic cystostomy was performed in France in 1560 by Pierre Franco

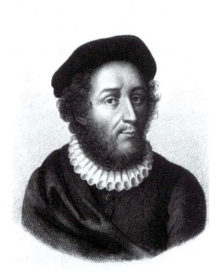

Figure 14: Guy de Chauliac (engraving, 14th century)

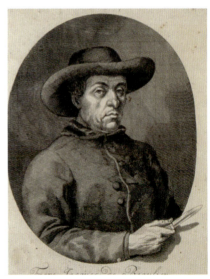

Figure 15: Jacques de Beaulieu (Berge, 1650).

(1502-1560). But as the results were disastrous, this technique was not employed again for almost two hundred years.

In 1697, Jacques de Beaulieu (1651-1714) (Fig. 15), better known under the name of "Frère Jacques" introduced a modification to perineal cystostomy. Instead of using a median incision, he performed a lateral one which brought better results because the haemorrhage was less abundant, the urethra was not traumatized and the healing of the wound was much faster.

The surgeon Jean Louis Petit (1674-1750), who described the anatomical triangle situated in the lumbar muscular region which is still named after him, invented the first curved catheter, which was built in 1700. This type of catheter was adapted to the normal anatomical direction of the male urethra and facilitated surgery for bladder stones.

Then came two surgeons, Henri Francois le Dran (1685-1770) and Jean Baseilhac (1703-1783) known as "Frère Côme", who between 1727 and 1755 brought the technique of the perineal and the suprapubic cystostomy to the highest degree of perfection attainable before the development of antiseptic and aseptic surgery. Frère Côme obtained an international reputation by his successful performances of cystostomies for stone extraction.

We also have to mention Claude Nicolas Le Cat (1700-1768) who worked in Rouen and developed the so called "taille laterale" type of cystotomy. These operations, brilliant as they were for this period, when performed by specialists, still continued to have disastrous results when performed by less skilful individuals. This is the reason which led some surgeons to search for a less complicated operation to remove stones from the bladder, and brought about the development of (endoscopic) lithotrity.

Urological surgery in France in the 19th Century

It was the improvements in the lithotripsy techniques during the 19th century which stimulated the real birth of urology during that century.[9] It is indeed in these years, that urological surgery began to be individualized as a specialty. In fact, during the 19th century the basic foundations of pathological, surgical and instrumental knowledge were established, which, in some cases, have undergone little changes up to our era of modern urology.

The first name to be noticed in the 19th century for his achievements in the field of urological surgery was the general surgeon Jean Civiale (1792-1867). (Fig. 16) In Paris, he performed on January 13, 1822, the very first lithotrity or minimal invasive blind crushing of a bladder stone. He performed the operation with an instrument called the "lithotriteur à archet" (bow lithotriptor), (Fig. 17) which consisted of four branches in-between which the stone was caught and crushed. He was also the first surgeon to specifically devote in 1824, a number of beds specifically to "urological patients" in the Hospital Necker in Paris. (Fig. 18)

The urological surgeon Jean Jacques Leroy d'Etiolles (1798-1860) (Fig. 19) was probably the one who designed the lithotriptor used by Civiale. Between 1822 and 1846 Leroy d'Etiolles presented several ameliorated models

[9] Kuss, R. and W. Gregoir. *Histoire illustrée de l'Urologie*, 1988.

based on his original concept. However he had to defend the intellectual property of this type of lithotriptor before the Academy of Sciences as he claimed that the instrument maker Charrière gave the instrument, Leroy's invention, to Civiale to use as a first in a patient.[10] First the claim was accepted, but later dismissed. Mystery remains who was in his rights. In 1834, Leroy d'Etiolles invented urethral explorators of different sizes, by means of which it was possible to estimate the calibre and the number of urethral strictures. He went further and was the first surgeon to develop an instrument to remove the prostatic adenoma through the urethra, by means of a cutting noose wire. With this development he was a pioneer in transurethral resection of the prostate.

In 1832, Charles Louis Heurteloup (1793-1864) invented the first real lithotripter with two branches sliding into one another, thus permitting the grasping of the stone, which was then crushed by percussion on the inner branch with a small hammer. Joseph Frederic Benoit Charrière (1803-1876) (Fig. 20) one year later perfected this instrument by the addition of a screw on the handle. Charrière was also the inventor of the "French" scale (Fig. 21) for measuring the size of catheters and instruments, that is still in use today.

In 1834, Louis Auguste Mercier (1811-1882) designed an elbowed-end catheter which also is still in use, without having been modified. In 1836, Auguste Nelaton (1807-1873) (Fig. 22) presented in cooperation with the Good Year Company a rubber catheter with a straight tip, which still bears his name.[11] In 1841, Louis Auguste Mercier was also the first

[10] Zykan, M. The relationship between the physician and the instrument maker. *De Historia Urologiae Europaeae*, vol 17, 139, 2010.

[11] Van Kerrebroeck, Ph. *The urinary bladder: problems and solutions*. 2010.

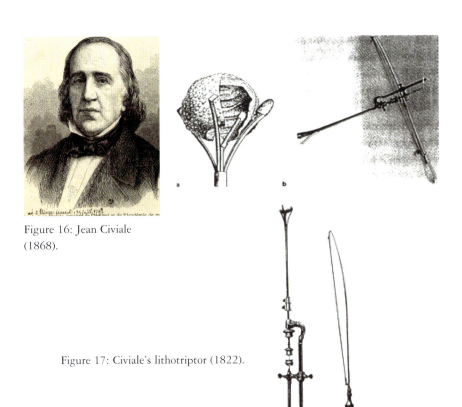

Figure 16: Jean Civiale (1868).

Figure 17: Civiale's lithotriptor (1822).

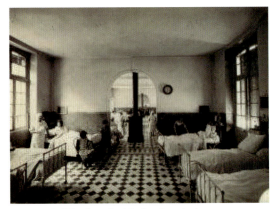

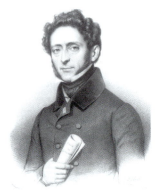

Figure 18: Ward at the Necker hospital.

Figure 19: Leroy d'Etiolles (Belliard after Viallot, 1855).

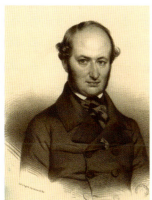

Figure 20: Jospeh Frederic Benoit Charrière

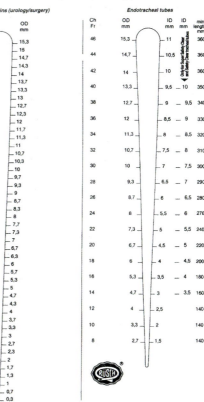

Figure 21: The French scale for catheters and tubes (Rusch).

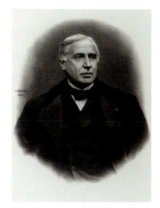

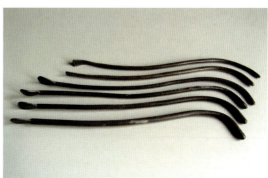

Figure 22: Auguste Nélaton.　　Figure 23: Set of beniqués.

to give a clear and precise description of the prostatic adenoma, with its median and lateral lobes and the role played by these lobes in the retention of urine, whether partial or complete.

Around the same time, Pierre Jules Beniqué (1809-1851) invented his metallic double-curved dilatators (Fig. 23) which are still utilized for the dilatation of urethral strictures. In 1826 Pierre Saloman Segalas d'Etcheparre (1792-1875) used for the first time a "speculum urethrocystoscopique" that allowed an initial form of urethrocystoscopy. However in 1853, Antoine Jean Desormeaux (1815-1894) (Fig. 24), although not the first urological surgeon to conceive the endoscopic exploration of the bladder, introduced the first practical cystoscope. In his "Traité de l'endoscopie" published in 1865, he described many aspects of the pathological

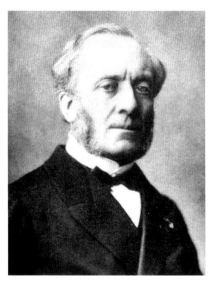

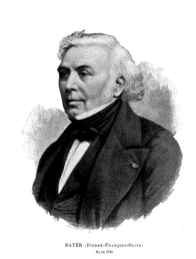

Figure 24: Antoine Jean Desormeaux.   Figure 25: Pierre François Olive Rayer.

bladder. However it is only with the Austrian urologist Nitze, who introduced his cystoscope in Vienna in 1879, that cystoscopy attained its real development.

Together with these technical developments, knowledge about the possible relation between dysfunction of the urinary tract and kidney function deterioration also became evident. In that respect we have to mention Pierre Francois Olive Rayer (1793-1867). (Fig. 25) He was a French physician who was a native of Saint Sylvain in the Calvados area and made important contributions in the fields of pathological anatomy, physiology, comparative pathology and parasitology.[12]

Rayer studied medicine in Caen, and after that in Paris at the Ecole Pratique des Hautes Etudes and at the Hôtel-Dieu. He became a physician at Hôpital Saint-Antoine (1825), and at the Hôpital de la Charité (1832), and was also a consultant-physician to King Louis-Philippe. In 1862 he attained the chair of comparative anatomy at the Faculty of Medicine of Paris. Between 1837 and 1841 he published a three-volume book on diseases of the kidney titled "Traité des maladies des reins", which introduced the concept of uropathy and was the foundation of clinical nephrology and uropathology in France.

In 1850 Jean Francois Reybard (1795-1851) performed for the first time an internal urethrotomy with a primitive urethrotome. (Fig. 26) In 1855, Jules Romain François Maisonneuve (1809-1897) (Fig. 27) used his urethrotome with a guide for internal section of urethral strictures and presented it to the

---

12
Caveribert, R. "La Vie et l'oeuvre de Rayer." *Th. Med.*, Paris, 1931.

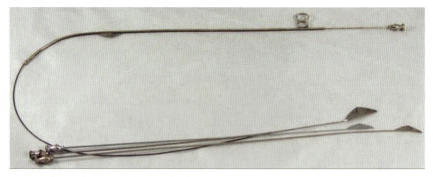

Figure 26: Urethrotome after Reybard.

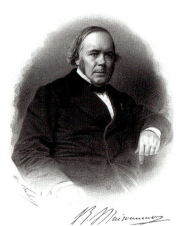

Figure 27: Jules Romain Maisonneuve

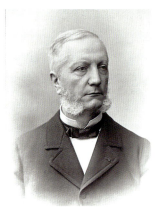

Figure 28: Jean Casimir Felix Guyon.

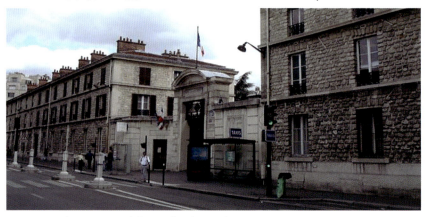

Figure 29: The entrance of the Necker hospital

Academy of Medicine. This urethrotome was so simple and so easy to manoeuvre, that actual models are still based on his original design.

All these personalities were general surgeons that practised urogenital surgery. In fact it was with the arrival of Jean Casimir Felix Guyon (1831-1920) at Necker Hospital in Paris, on July 9, 1867, that urology started to undergo so many improvements, that it really could claim its own place among the surgical specialties. A place it has held since then.

The birth of Urology

Jean Casimir Félix Guyon (21 July 1831 – 2 August 1920) (Fig. 28) was born on Ile-Bourbon (Réunion).[13] He studied medicine in Paris, receiving his doctorate in 1858. He was appointed médecin des hôpitaux in 1864 and became successor to Civiale in 1867 with a specific interest in the urinary tract. In 1877 he was appointed as a professor of surgical pathology. However he was such a pioneer in the field of genito-urinary surgery and he was so devoted to the study of the problems of the urinary tract and their treatment, that his teaching was recognized officially by the University of Paris. He became in 1890, the first professor of Genito-urinary Surgery at the University of Paris. As such he can be considered to have been the first professor of urology worldwide. In 1878 he became a member of the Académie de Médecine. At Hôpital Necker he held clinics that were attended also by students from many foreign countries and that were received with great enthousiasm.[14] (Fig.29)

Felix Guyon can definitely be called the father of modern urology. The German urolo-

---

13
Haas, L.F. "Felix Guyon 1831–1920". *Journal of Neurology, Neurosurgery & Psychiatry* 74 (6): 698, 2003.

14
N.N., *La clinique urologique de Necker*, 1912–1933. Paris, Masson. 1933.

gist Israel said at an international meeting of urologists held in 1910 that, "all the urologists of the world were his pupils", as he was the first surgeon to give all of his life to the development and to the scientific improvement of urology. In 1896 Guyon founded the Association Française d'Urologie and in 1907, he along with urologists from Europe, the United States and South America established the Association Internationale d'Urologie.

Guyon was president of this Association from 1907 till 1914. The Association changed his name in 1919 into the Societé Internationale d'Urologie (SIU) as it still exists today. In 1979 he was commemorated on a postage stamp, issued by France at the occasion of the 18th Congress of the SIU, held in Paris (Fig. 30). The Hôpital Félix Guyon, located in Saint-Denis, Réunion, is named in his honour and in Paris also a street bears his name. (Fig. 31)

Although he was primarily known for work with genitourinary anatomy, Guyon is credited with the discovery of the ulnar canal at the wrist, that is now indicated as Guyon's

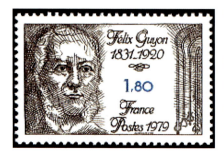

Figure 30: A stamp with Guyon's portrait.

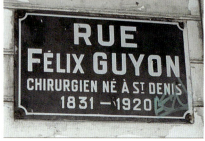

Figure 31: The Felix Guyon street in Paris.

canal. Ulnar nerve compression at this location is sometimes referred to as "Guyon's tunnel syndrome". However his greatest contributions are in the field of urology. He described the clinical symptoms of superficial and infiltrating cancer of the bladder. He gave a very definite description of bladder distension and its repercussion on the kidneys, and also analysed very precisely the subsequent intoxication caused by the rising of urea in the blood.

His clinical studies on prostate cancer are still classics. He made important contributions to the physiology of the contractions of the normal and of the pathological bladder and was also recognized during nearly thirty years as the master of lithotrity. His mortality rate in this special operation never rose above 2%.

Guyon also established definitely the technique of internal urethrotomy, by setting an indwelling-catheter in the urethra following the operation. With this amelioration, he brought down the mortality rate of this operation from 60% to 2%! He gave a complete clinical description of urinary septicaemia. He also described the best way to perform bi-manual palpation of the kidneys. He brought the technique of suprapubic cystostomy to such a degree of perfection that we still perform this operation in accordance with it.

Guyon also proposed the two-stage operation in traumatic ruptures of the urethra in cases where there is extensive injury to adjoining tissues. All of his conceptions were clearly set forth in the book he wrote on clinical urology, entitled "Leçons cliniques", which for many years was considered the bible of urology.

He was also a pioneer in modern research technique as he was a protagonist in translational research. He promoted the connection between clinical experience and observations at the bed of the patient and experimental findings based on laboratory research.

Guyon also founded an eminent school of urologists around him, based on his interest in teaching and training. Therefore he can be considered not only as the first urologist but also as the first complete and global urologist combining clinical work, research, teaching and management "avant la lettre" and all this in an international perspective.

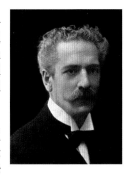

Figure 32: Joaquin Albarran.

French Urologists in the 19th century and the beginning of the 20th century

The work of Guyon in Paris stimulated many young and bright doctors to start training in urology under his guidance. One of them was **Joaquin Albarran** (1860-1912), full name Joaquin Albarrán Maria y Dominguez.[15] (Fig. 32) He was born in Cuba, but went to Paris at the age of 18, where he worked and studied under many renowned physicians. Albarran regarded the anatomist Louis-Antoine Ranvier (1835–1922) and the urologist Jean Casimir Félix Guyon as major influences in his career.

Albarran started his training in urology with Guyon in 1883 and became his most beloved pupil and collaborator. In 1906, after the retirement of Guyon, he was appointed to succeed him as director of the Clinic of Urology at the Hôpital Necker and he continued the work of his master. Although his career was very short, his scientific achievements equalled, if not surpassed, those of his predecessor. Albarran's

15
Casey, R.G. and J. Thornhill. "Joaquin Maria Albarran Y Dominguez: microbiologist, histologist, and urologist, a lifetime from orphan in Cuba to Nobel nominee." *Int J Urol.* 13(9):1159-61, 2006.

early career was spent in the fields of microbiology and histopathology, but he later switched to urology where he made several important contributions.

He was the first French physician to perform a perineal prostatectomy. He was a three-time winner of the Goddard Prize, and was nominated in 1912 for a Nobel Prize in Medicine. Albarran although a Cuban by birth, was French by adoption and it was in Paris that he received his whole medical education and that all his achievements were made. He gave such an impulse to clinical urology that most of his observations are still up-to-date.

In 1888, he described the role played by the colon bacilli in the infections of the urinary tract. Four years later, he explained the mechanism of the formation of hydronephrosis, and made an elaborate study of perinephritis, showing that this could be of two types, that is, consecutive to a renal infection or to a generalized infection. The year 1897 saw the greatest achievement of Albarran, the adaptation of a cystoscopic lever to a Nitze cystoscope, which rendered possible the catheterization of the ureters and thus opened the way to complete exploration of the urinary tract. This device was to become known as the Albarran lever.

In 1898, he described the pathology of the urinary abscess and the role played by anaerobes in this type of fulminating infection. Two years later, he published his histo-pathological findings on the pathological prostate and showed that benign hypertrophy was in reality the hypertrophy of the peri-urethral glands of the prostatic urethra, and that prostatic carcinoma had its origin in the prostate gland itself. In 1901, he established the final points in the technique of perineal prostatectomy and in 1908, he was able to publish his first hundred cases with only 2% mortality! In 1902 he gave the first clear description of tumours of the kidney and of the pelvis, and also showed the different ways by which the kidney could be infected by tuberculosis.

In 1905, Albarran demonstrated the excellent results obtained by early nephrectomy in renal tuberculosis and in the same year he promulgated the first physiological laws concerning the elimination of urea by the kidneys. Finally in 1909, three years before his death, he published a volume on genito-urinary surgery entitled "Medecine operatoire des voies urinaires", which was the completion of his brilliant career, and still stands as one of the greatest urological documents.

Even if Albarran was so important, we may not forget the achievements of other French urologists from the 19th century, who also contributed largely to the advancement of the speciality.[16]

Theodore Tuffier (1857-1929) demonstrated in 1887 the possibility of nephrectomy, by showing that the remaining kidney had enough capacity of compensation to allow a normal life, after that operation. He also demonstrated that a nephrostomy could be performed without any danger as long as momentary compression was applied to the renal vascular pedicle. He also established the best technique to suture an incision on the kidney itself. A few years later, he described capsular

16

Fischer, I. *Biographisches Lexikon der hervorragenden Ärzte der letzten fünfzig Jahre.* Berlin, Urban & Schwarzenberg, 1937.

nephropexy and also the best way to open the ureter and suture it afterwards, in order to avoid urinary fistulas, thus opening the way to the surgery of the ureter.

In the same year 1887, **Octave Pasteau** (1870-1957) introduced the graduated ureteral catheter thus enabling the operator to know exactly to what distance the catheter is introduced in the ureter.

Albarran, outside of his great personal achievements, contributed by his teaching to the scientific training of many urologists who continued his work. Among these were Legueu, Luys, Chevassu, Heitz-Boyer, Papin, Jeanbrau, Lepoutre and Marion, who were the most important urologists to follow in the steps of Guyon and Albarran.

In 1913, **Felix Legueu** (1863-1939) (Fig. 33) was appointed Professor of Urology and started where Albarran had left off. Legueu was a clinical professor in Paris, and worked as urologist at Hôpital Necker. He was a member of the Académie de Médecine. He was responsible for the transition of French urology to the 20th century. Among his main achievements were the establishment of surgical indications in the surgery of renal lithiasis, and the application of local anaesthesia to prostatectomy, thus enabling urologists to operate on patients who could not have survived the postoperative complications of general anaesthesia which was not so well developed yet.

Legueu also made great contributions to the study of the renal secretion, to the surgical treatment of urethral strictures and to the sur-

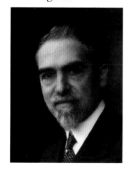

Figure 33:
Felix Legueu.

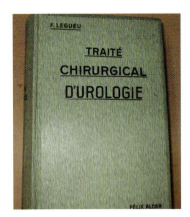

Figure 34:
"Traite chirurgical d'Urologie" by Legueu.

A TREATISE
ON
CYSTOSCOPY AND URETHROSCOPY

BY

DR. GEORGES LUYS

FORMER INTERNE, HOSPITALS OF PARIS; FORMER ASSISTANT IN THE DEPARTMENT OF URINARY DISEASES AT THE LARIBOISIERE HOSPITAL; LAUREATE OF THE FACULTY OF THE ACADEMY OF MEDICINE.

TRANSLATED AND EDITED WITH ADDITIONS

BY

ABR. L. WOLBARST, M.D.,
NEW YORK

CYSTOSCOPIST, BETH ISRAEL HOSPITAL; CONSULTING UROLOGIST, CENTRAL ISLIP AND MANHATTAN STATE HOSPITALS; GENITO-URINARY SURGEON, WEST SIDE GERMAN DISPENSARY AND HOSPITAL; AUTHOR OF "GONORRHEA IN THE MALE," ETC.

WITH 217 FIGURES IN THE TEXT AND 24 CHROMOTYPOGRAPHIC PLATES OUTSIDE THE TEXT, INCLUDING 76 DRAWINGS FROM ORIGINAL WATER COLORS.

ST. LOUIS
C. V. MOSBY COMPANY
1918

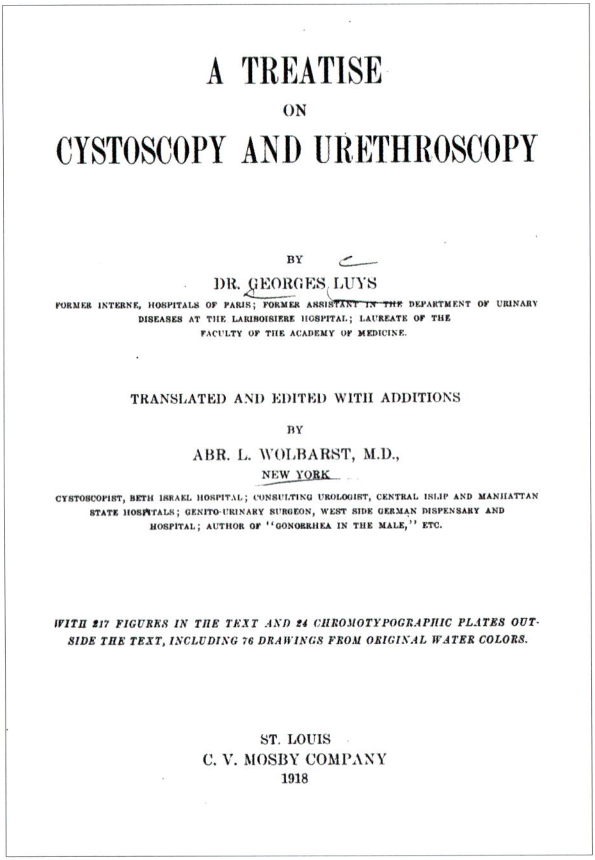

Figure 35:
A Treatise on Cystoscopy and Urethroscopy by G. Luys.

gery of the ruptured urethra. His book, entitled "Traité chirurgical d' Urologie" and published in 1910 was the completion of his master's publications. (Fig. 34) In 1913 he described a procedure for the closure of a vesicovaginal fistula, an operative technique, indicated as the "Dittel-Forgue-Legueu operation", named after Legueu together with **Leopold von Dittel** (1815-1898) and **Émile Forgue** (1860-1943). A few surgical instruments bear Legueu's name, such as the "Legueu bladder retractor" and the "Legueu bladder spatula". Legueu died in his home from carbon monoxide poisoning.

The procedure of filling the bladder with air in order to be examined was popularized in France around 1905 by the Parisian urologist **George Luys** (1870-1953), who apparently imitated the Valentine urethroscope and equipped it with an aspirating tube. (Fig. 35) Luys started with electrocoagulation in 1913-1914. From this year on, he employed the "forage de la prostate," inducing coagulation necrosis in the prostate via a coil-shaped electrode. An air pump unfolded the bladder and posterior urethra. He used a cystoscope which had a bulb-tipped electrode (this part being the cauterising part) on the end. He reportedly achieved satisfactory results in more than 90% of his patients. His method was used mainly in France and Germany.

By 1926, Luys reported on over 100 electro-surgical operations for prostatic hypertrophy. Luys is also considered one of the earliest to achieve separate urine collection by catheterizing urine directly from the ureters. He also created various modified designs of equipment. The most important models included adjustable forceps and scopes with improved aspiration channels. He also made the practice of urine separation a popular methodology. He modified the Valentine model for men and women, going so far as to perform some modest operative procedures with it, such as cauterizing bladder tumours and the prostate.

Luys was also a master in removing foreign bodies from the bladder with a small forceps. He also improved and extended the cystoscope, creating further therapeutic uses such as new methods for treating prostate conditions.

Overall, Luys was important for further expanding urethroscopy and cystoscopy in France. In 1914 he took Young's method and applied it to prostate obstruction operations, also under direct visualization. Luys seems to have modified it somewhat by changing the exact method of placement of the cystoscope. Luys recognized it as a minimally invasive procedure, speaking of how it was superior to the "gravity" of a transvesical (open) procedure. Strangely, despite Luys's success, it appears that open prostatectomies still remained the procedure of choice in France till much later in the 20th century.

Maurice Chevassu (1877-1957) worked as a urologist in the Hopital Cochin in Paris. He is mostly known for the classification of tumours of the testicles which he published in 1906. He was also the first urologist to apply to urinary surgery the laws of Ambard who established the relation existing between the blood urea and the urea in the urine. Chevassu also contributed largely to the study of ureteropyelography.

Considered to be the most beloved pupil of Albarran, **Maurice Heitz-Boyer** (1876-1950) was the first urologist to practise electro-coagulation of superficial carcinomas of the bladder through the cystoscope. He achieved a breakthrough for endo-urology at the time by becoming one of the first to use high frequency treatment of prostate adenoma in 1911. He designed his own high frequency instrument and by 1921 his instruments had three different optical systems and also three different electrodes. Heitz-Boyer had visited the American pioneer Young in Baltimore, who had demonstrated his punch operation. It was apparently Heitz-Boyer who advised Young to use high-frequency current and was apparently surprised that he was not using it.

Edmond Papin (1876-1951), another disciple of Albarran, contributed largely to the improvement of Volker's and Lichtenberg's pyelography introduced in 1906. His greatest achievement though, was his study of the congenital malformations of the kidneys and ureters. He also published his observations on hydronephrosis, based on dynamic images of retrograde pyelography. To surgical urology he brought new techniques of pyelotomy and of hemi-nephrectomy, and he introduced the denervation of the kidneys.

Further development of urological departments was slow outside Paris. However after World War I the interest in the pathology of the lower urinary tract increased and specific specialist (urologists) were appointed in other centres in France although mainly in University Centres.

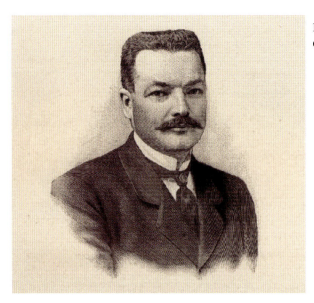

Figure 36: Georges Marion.

Emile Alexis Jeanbrau (1873-1950), created the first Department of Urology at the University of Montpellier in 1908 and became the first professor of Urology in Montpellier in 1922. He made a large contribution to the diagnosis and treatment of ureteral stones.

Carlos Lepoutre (1882-1950), was the first professor of Urology at the University of Lille, and made an important study on the ruptured urethra. His book entitled "Les ruptures de l'urèthre" was published in 1934. With Edmond Pillet of Rouen he was the first urologist to promote the palpation of the kidney in the vertical position and also the making of pyelograms in this position. Lepoutre also published two books on Surgical Urology.

Louis Ombredanne (1871-1956), although not a urologist but a paediatric and plastic surgeon, has developed two important urological techniques, one for the cure of penile hypospadias on children and the other for scrotal orchidopexy in cases of ectopy of the testicle. Another surgeon, **Simon-Emmanuel Duplay** (1836-1924) also introduced a technique which is still employed sometimes for the cure of hypospadias. Together with the German surgeon **Karl Thiersch** (1822-1895), his name is associated with an operation for repair of distal hypospadias, the so called Thiersch-Duplay technique.[17]

We cannot finish a review of urology in France in the 19th century and early 20th century without mentioning one the greatest disciple of Guyon and Albarran who was an outstanding master of French urology. His name is **Georges Marion** (1869-1960).[18] (Fig. 36) He headed the Department of Urology at Lariboisière Hospital in Paris from 1908 to 1931 and then the same department at Necker Hospital after he was appointed Professor of Urology at the University of Paris.

Marion's publications are numerous. His main ones are his "Precis de therapeutique urinaire" published in 1910, his "Leçons de chirurgie urinaire", published in 1912, and a few years later, his "Traité pratique de cystoscopie et de catheterisme ureteral", which he wrote in collaboration with Heitz-Boyer, and which was the first of its kind to be published in the world. This manual has been at the base of the teaching of different aspects of pathological conditions of the bladder observed through the cystoscope.

In 1921 he published his "Traité d'Urologie" in two volumes which has been re-edited many times, and is surely one of the best

---

[17] Pagel, J. *Biographical Dictionary of excellent doctors of the nineteenth century.* Berlin, 1901.

[18] Nezhot, P. *History of Endoscopy.* Online: chapter 15, www.laparaoscopy.blogs.com, 2012.

books on urology of that time. This manual has been written by Marion alone and, besides being an interesting scientific book, it is a pleasure to read because of his eloquent style. He also published in 1936 a book entitled "Quelques verités premières en urologie". Marion, apart from being a marvellous teacher, has created many new surgical techniques some of which are still used today. He developed an "enlarged pyelotomy" in which the incision includes both the pelvis and the renal parenchyma and permitted to remove large stones from the kidney easily and with no danger. He also promoted a new technique for nephrostomies for drainage of the kidney, with the use of Tripier's dilatation conductor.

His greatest gift to renal surgery was the management of the renal vascular pedicle during nephrectomy, when the latter is torn off, or slips. He was known for his demonstration of this technique by purposely tearing away the renal pedicle and then show what to do in such a case to control the haemorrhage and save the patient's life. Marion also contributed greatly to the amelioration of the postoperative treatment following prostatectomy, with the different drainage tubes he has devised. In 1913, he developed his own technique for the resection of bladder diverticula.

A few years later he described his own technique for the transvesical surgical cure of vesico-vaginal fistula, a technique which, if well-followed, enabled one to obtain a very high cure rate. He also published a very elegant technique for the cure of female stress urinary incontinence, by shortening the urethral sphincter. Marion also contributed largely to the surgery of the urethra and in this field his circular urethroraphy is still used sometimes for the treatment of traumatic rupture of the posterior urethra. Finally Marion also devised an elegant technique for the surgical cure of hypospadias.

With Marion, the heritage of the 19th century passes into the modern era of the 20th century urology. But for sure, actual urological practice owes a lot to these inventive and original predecessors from the 19th century.

Urology in France in the 19th Century

It is obvious that many achievements have been brought to us by the French School of Urology as initiated in the 19th century. These contributions are so numerous and so important that it is possible to say that no other country in Europe has done so much for our specialty. Lithotripsy has a long history in France but developed over the centuries from primitive lithotrity techniques by semi-doctors and with a very high mortality to modern techniques of lithotripsy applied by specialist surgeons called since the end of the 19th century "urologists".

During the 19th century, many technical innovations in the field of urology, helpfull and usefull in endoscopic procedures as well as in open surgical procedures on the uro-genital tract, were developed and clinically tested in France. Many of these techniques are still applied worldwide today. Also the semiology of the uro-genital tract was ameliorated as it was progressively based on scientific data, making urology a scientific discipline but still with a strong input from history taking, clinical symptoms and physical examination. Several innovative diagnostic modalities, still practised today, were established at that time.

Urology developed as a separate specialty within the field of surgery in France at the end of the 19th century, starting with specifically dedicated beds. In the course of that century, urological surgeons developed into urologists and were slowly recognised as such by their peers. Initially urology was developed in Paris but later also spread to other, mainly university centres throughout the country. The general surgeon with interest in genito-urinary surgery, Jean Civiale paved the way to urology and the genito-urinary surgeon Casimir Guyon established urology as a separate specialty.

Furthermore the international acceptance of urology as a separate speciality was pioneered by French urologists at the end of the 19th century. At the same time, urology developed in France as a global speciality with interest in anatomy, physiology and pathology. These developments were the basis for the excellence of French urologists since then, but also allowed for urology to develop as a global, clinical and also scientific specialty worldwide.

Correspondence to:
Prof. P.E.V. Van Kerrebroeck
Maastricht University Medical Center
Dept. of Urology
PO Box 5800
NL- 6202 AZ Maastricht
The Netherlands

RENÉ KÜSS (1913-2006) - A TRANSPLANT PIONEER IN PARIS

Dirk Schultheiss[1], Alain Jardin[2]

1. Department of Urology, Protestant Hospital, Giessen, Germany.

2. 9 Boulevard du Temple, 75003 Paris, France

Introduction

Many of the crucial innovations that would facilitate kidney transplantation have been made in France. The initial impulse came from the surgical school in Lyon, where Alexis Carrel (1873-1944), under the guidance of Mathieu Jaboulay (1860-1913), introduced modern vascular anastomosis with sutures in 1902, which 10 years later earned Carrel the Nobel Prize in medicine. In 1906 Jaboulay tried to graft animal kidneys to the elbows of two patients and Carrel performed a successful autotransplantation in a dog in 1908.

After World War I, Serge Voronoff (1866-1951), a French surgeon of Russian origin, performed a variety of transplantation experiments in his research laboratory at the College de France and later became famous with his doubtful rejuvenation technique of transplanting testicular tissue. From 1950 on, Paris became one of the world's leading centres for kidney transplantation, mainly through the achievements of the urological surgeon René Küss (1913-2006) and the nephrologist Jean Hamburger (1909-1992) from the Necker Hospital. They played a pivotal role for French nephrology by performing the first hemodialysis in France in 1955 and by contributing to modern transplantation immunology.[1,2]

A career in urological surgery

René Küss was born in Paris on May 3,

---

[1] Starzl, T.E. "The French heritage in clinical transplantation." *Transplant Rev* (Orlando) 7:65, 1993.

[2] Jardin, A. "Renal transplantation." In: J.J. Mattelaer and D. Schultheiss, eds. *Europe – the cradle of Urology*. European Association of Urology: Arnhem, 2010. 237-243.

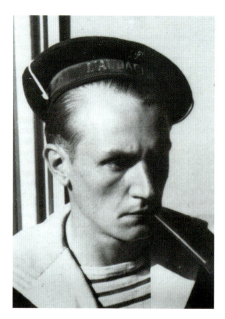

Figure 1: René Küss around 1937 (Archive Prof. Alain Jardin).

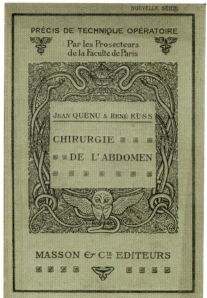

Figure 2a: *"Chirurgie de l'abdomen"* from 1949.

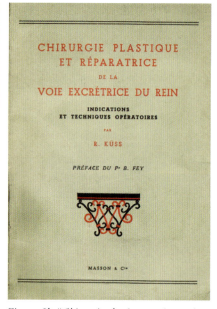

Figure 2b: *"Chirurgie plastique et réparatrice de la voie excrétrice du rein"* from 1954.

1913, the son of the surgeon Georges Küss (1877-1967), who was a master of hypogastric prostatectomy. The elder Küss allowed his son to get acquainted with medical practice at an early age, with René visiting an operating theatre for the first time at the age of seven. Later, René Küss started his surgical training as a young student at the department of Robert Proust (1873-1935), brother of the famous writer Marcel Proust. In 1900 Robert Proust, at that time under the guidance of Félix Guyon (1831-1920) and Joaquin Albarrán (1860-1912), had published his landmark medical thesis on perineal prostatectomy, a procedure which in France was called *"proustatectomie."*

In 1939 Küss became *"interne des Hôpitaux de Paris"* and he soon entered military service as a surgeon in World War II. (Fig. 1) He survived the attack on the French fleet at Mers-El-Kébir, on the coast of French Algeria, when the ship he served on was sunk. Later he led the surgical team of General Patton's 3rd American Army and participated with the French Resistance in the liberation of Paris in 1945.

After the war, Küss dedicated his career to urology. He first worked at the Cochin Hospital in Paris, until he created a multi-hospital department of urology at Foch Hospital, St. Louis Hospital and later Pitié-Salpêtrière Hospital, all in Paris.[3,4,5]

Among his early textbooks on surgery and surgical urology are *Chirurgie de l'abdomen* (Fig. 2a) from 1949, together with Jean Quénu (1889-1975)[6] and *Chirurgie plastique et réparatrice de la voie excrétrice du rein* (Fig. 2b) from 1954.[7]

3
Cinqualbre, J. and B.D. Kahan. "René Küss: Fifty years of retroperitoneal placement of renal transplants." *Transplant Proc* 34: 3019, 2002.

4
Charpentier, B. "Laudatio to Professor René Küss." *Transpl Int* 19:770, 2006.

5
Chatelain, C. "Eulogy of M. René Küss." *Bull Acad Natl Med.* 192:469, 2008.

6
Quénu, J. and R. Küss. *Chirurgie de l'abdomen.* Masson: Paris, 1949.

7
Küss, R. *Chirurgie plastique et réparatrice de la voie excrétrice du rein.* Masson: Paris, 1954.

René Küss served the Société Internationale d'Urologie (SIU) as General Secretary from 1952 until 1979, and as President from 1979 until 1985. In 1971, Küss founded the "Société Francaise de Transplantation," the first scientific society dedicated to transplantation medicine in Europe. Beside many honours and titles, Küss was also president of the French College of Surgeons Meeting in 1980, and of the Académie Nationale de Médicine in 1987 and was awarded the EAU's Willy Gregoir Medal in 2002. Küss died on June 20, 2006.[3]

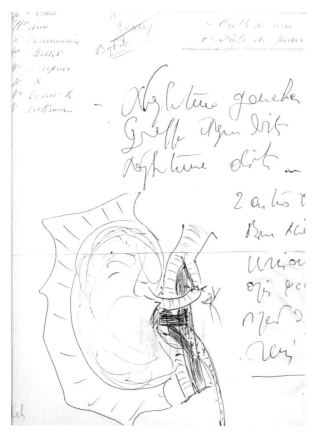

Figure 3: Operating protocol sketch outlined by René Küss with representation of the iliac retroperitoneal positioning of the kidney transplant with end-to-end internal iliac arterial anastomosis (dated November 6, 1960).

Kidney transplantation in Paris

With the introduction of successful hemodialysis with an "artificial kidney" by the Dutch nephrologist Willem Kolff (1911-2009) in 1944, there was an increasing interest in and new possibilities for the treatment of acute and chronic renal insufficiency. A first homograft on a young man was carried out unsuccessfully in 1945 at the Brigham Hospital in Boston. The same clinic succeeded in transplantation of a kidney among homozygote twins in 1954, which is considered the first successful living donor kidney transplantation, worldwide. There were many similar efforts in the decade between, which often ended in disappointments.

After the war René Küss, together with several other surgeons in Paris, actively engaged in vascular surgery and transplantation of the kidney. They performed several animal experiments in 1948. Following another report of a short-term success of cadaveric donor kidney transplantation in Chicago in June 1950, these three surgical teams in Paris, guided by Küss and two cardiac surgeons, Charles Dubost (1914-1991) and Marceau Servelle (1912-2002), started a series of operations themselves.

The organs were either taken from living donors, or from prisoners sentenced to death who had agreed on having their kidneys removed soon after decapitation. In January 1951 the first transplantations were performed at Broussais Hospital (Debost) and at Cochin Hospital (Küss). It was with these operations that Küss perfected the retroperitoneal placement of the donor kidney into the iliac fossa and anastomosis to the iliac vessels, which to this day remains the standard kidney transplantation procedure. (Fig. 3)

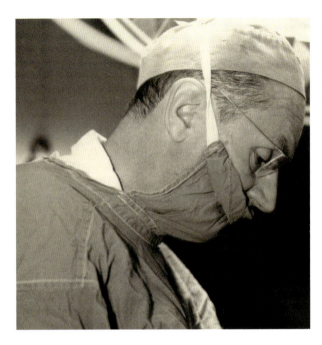

Figure 4: René Küss in the operating theatre in 1978 (Archive Prof. Alain Jardin).

After a series of eight unsuccessful operations (five performed by Küss himself) the team decided to abandon this operation, and Küss summarised in 1952: "...in the present state of knowledge, the only rational transplantation would be an exchange between monozygotic twins." This was then the rare case of the abovementioned milestone transplantation at Brigham Hospital in 1954. Following these disappointing attempts Küss focused on plastic and reconstructive surgery of the urinary tract and he perfected techniques for ureteral anastomosis that would later be useful for establishing routine kidney transplantation in the 1960's.

Only with the introduction of an immunosuppressive regimen did Küss again enter the field of transplantation. He performed a series of six living donor operations at Foch Hospital in 1961 and 1962, where the recipients were initially treated with total body irradiation and later administered steroids and the new drug 6-mercaptopurine for immunosuppression. Küss continued his pioneering work in transplantation surgery for years and received many awards for his work.[8] (Fig. 4)

Art connoisseur and collector

René Küss had been introduced to the world of art by his father and built up a huge and outstanding collection of paintings during his life. Since 1933, he had been attracted to the city of Honfleur at the northwestern coast of France, where the artists Gustave Courbet, Eugène Boudin and Claude Monet had formed the *école de Honfleur* (Honfleur school) which later on helped give birth to the impressionist movement. Küss befriended contemporary French painters and became engaged in the "Société des Artistes honfleurais."

Besides collecting old masters like Cranach, Rubens, Watteau, and Tiepolo, his private collection of paintings also consisted of works from Boudin, Jongkind, Toulouse-Lautrec, Vuillard, Sisley, Gauguin, Renoir, Rouault, Bonnard, and Monet. Küss was especially proud to have won the bidding battle against the actress Liz Taylor at an auction in Paris in 1957 for the painting "Trouville. Docks at low tide (1892-96)" painted by Eugene Boudin. (Fig. 5) After the death of Küss, his collection was auctioned by Christie's in Paris and London in December 2006.[4,5,9]

Sportsman and "Automobiliste"

René Küss was an active sportsman involved in tennis, football, swimming, skiing,

8
Küss, R. "Human renal transplantation memories, 1951 to 1981," in: P.I. Terasaki (ed). *History of Transplantation: Thirty-Five Recollections.* UCLA Tissue Typing Laboratory: Los Angeles, 1991. 37–59.

9
Christie's: "Collection du Professeur René Küss." Auction catalogue. Christie's : Paris, 2006.

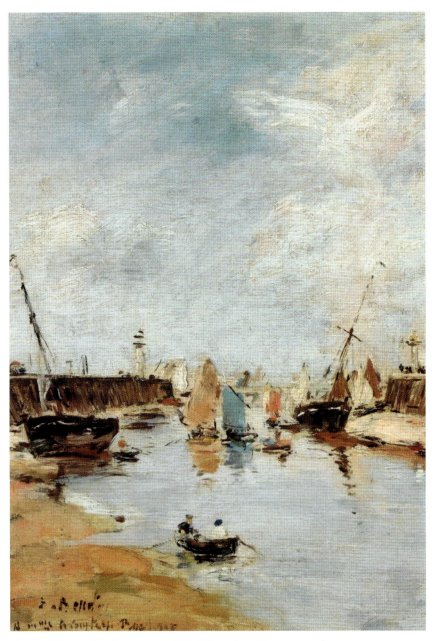

Figure 5: Eugene Boudin, "Trouville. Docks at low tide", 1892-96.

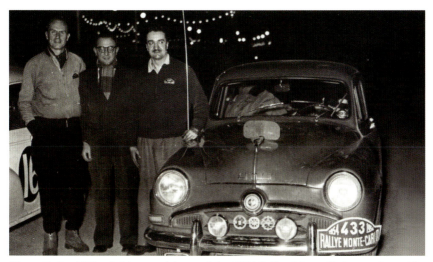

Figure 6: René Küss (left) as participant of the 1954 Rallye Monte Carlo together with his close friends the radiologist F. Degand and the venerologist A. Siboulet (Archive Prof. Alain Jardin).

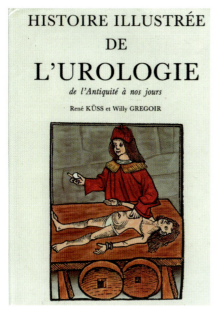

Figure 7a:"*Histoire illustrée de l' urologie de l'Antiquité a nos jours*" from 1989.

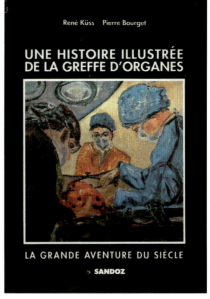

Figure 7b:"*Une histoire illustrée de la greffe d'organes*" from 1992.

and horse riding. Moreover he had a passion for hunting and car races. In 1954 he participated in the Rallye Monte Carlo together with his close friend the venerologist André Siboulet and finished the race with a good final result. [5] (Fig. 6)

Medical historian

During the last two decades of his life René Küss was also engaged in the field of medical history and published two extensive books: *Histoire illustrée de l'urologie de l'Antiquité a nos jours* (Fig. 7a) in 1989, together with the urologist Willy Gregoir (1920-2000),[10] and *Une histoire illustrée de la greffe d'organes* (Fig. 7b) in 1992 together with the medical journalist Pierre Bourget.[11]

10
Küss, R. and W. Gregoir. *Histoire illustrée de l' urologie de l'Antiquité a nos jours.* Les Éditions Roger Dacosta : Paris, 1989.

11
Küss, R. and P. Bourget. *Une histoire illustrée de la greffe d'organes.* Rueil-Malmaison : Sandoz, 1992.

Correspondence to:
Prof. Dr. med. Dirk Schultheiss
Chairman, History Office, European Association of Urology (EAU)
Department of Urology, Protestant Hospital,
Paul-Zipp-Str. 171, 35398 Giessen, Germany
Email: dirk.schultheiss@urologie-giessen.de

THE AUTHOR RESPONDS: CORRECTIONS TO VOLUME 19

Corrections to article: „Urology in Lwów, Lemberg and Lviv: how political changes influenced the development of medicine and urology. Stanisław Laskownicki (1892-1978)-the first professor of urology in Poland" in de Historia Urologiae Europaeae volume 19:

Page 60, line 14 from foot: for 1902, read 1899
Page 64, line 16 from top: for 1917, read 1899
Page 66, line 1 from foot: for 1917, read 1899

Additional References:

Page 65, 31 Borys, Y.B. Autobiography (2011).
Page 69, 32 Lesnyak, O.M. Personal reports (2011).

Commentary, remarks

In the post-Soviet era, the Ukrainian system of healthcare and academically education are completely differs from the Western one. In Ukraine the goals of Medical University are to teach students and conduct postgraduate education of the physicians. Only few Ukrainian Medical Universities have their own Clinics with beds. In Lviv, there are not university clinics. Department of Urology is based at hospitals. In these hospitals there are offices, they have the staff and manager. For example Medical University of Lviv has 20% of beds in the Department of the Urology of Lviv Regional Clinical Hospital.

In the history of medicine, the important developments are mostly reduced to a single person's work and ideas. However, such important developments can rarely be reduced only to the heads of the departments or the institutes. The special regulation and situation in urological service in Lviv shows that also many other top urologists have contributed to modernisation of the urology in the city in last two decades. Not only, the heads of the department of urology but also their associates and co-worker have enormous contributed to the urology. Especially, it is worth to mention some of the chiefs of the urological units in Lviv who done it, namely under others doctors, associate professors and professors: Mykola Artyshchuk, Roman Sheremeta, Oleksandr Vladislavovich Shulyak and Andryi Cezarovich Borzhyievsky have credited to improve our speciality there.

Acknowledgements

Prof. Cezar Kaytanovich Borzhyiewsky, Prof. Yuryi B. Borys, Dr. Bohdan Y. Borys, Dr. Oleg M. Lesnyak and Prof. Oleksandr V. Shulyak.

Correspondence to:
Dr. T. Zajaczkowski
Klaus-Groth-Str. 16
D-45472 Muelheim an der Ruhr, Germany
Email: th.zajaczkowski@gmx.de

CONTENTS of VOLUME 1
de Historia Urologiae Europaeae
(1994)

FOREWORD by F.M.J. Debruyne	7
THE HISTORY OF THE EUROPEAN ASSOCIATION OF UROLOGY *by W. Grégoir*	9
THE HISTORY OF VENEREAL DISEASE *by J.J. Mattelaer*	55
ON THE EXCISION OF STONES BOTH ABOVE AND BELOW THE PUBIC BONE *by J.H. Francken and translated by M.A. Van Andel*	77
THE STRUCTURE OF THE KIDNEY FROM ARISTOTLE TO MALPIGHI *by S. Musitelli, H. Jallous, T. de Basiani and P. Marandola*	121
THE STRUCTURE AND THE FUNCTION OF THE TESTICLES FROM ARISTOTLE TO THE "TESTIS EXAMINATUS" OF CLAUDIUS AUBRY (1658) *by S. Musitelli, H. Jallous, T. de Basiani and P. Marandola*	131
THE HISTORY OF EXSTROPHY OF THE BLADDER: THE DUTCH CONTRIBUTION *by J.D.M. De Vries and J.B.D.M. Van Gool*	145
THE HISTORY OF SPINA BIFIDA *by J.B.D.M. Van Gool and J.D.M. De Vries*	153

CONTENTS of VOLUME 2
de Historia Urologiae Europaeae
(1995)

FOREWORD by F.M.J. Debruyne	7
INTRODUCTION by J.J. Mattelaer	9
THE HISTORY OF UROLOGY IN THE BRITISH ISLES by J. Blandy	11
THE HISTORY OF UROLOGY IN RUSSIA by L. Gorilovski	23
THE HISTORY OF UROLOGY IN AUSTRIA by H. Haschek	35
THE HISTORY OF UROLOGY IN ITALY by S. Musitelli, M. Pavone Macaluso, P. Marandola, M. Lamartina, H. Jallous, G.B. Ingargiola and A. Speroni	57
THE HISTORY OF UROLOGY IN BELGIUM by J.J. Mattelaer, W. Grégoir, A. Similon and J. De Leval	85
THE HISTORY OF UROLOGY IN POLAND by L.J. Mazurek	125
UROLOGICAL KNOWLEDGE IN RENAISSANCE SPAIN by R. Vela Navarrete	139
THE HISTORY OF UROLOGY IN SWEDEN by E. Lindstedt	159
THE HISTORY OF UROLOGY IN HUNGARY by P. Magasi	175

CONTENTS of VOLUME 3
de Historia Urologiae Europaeae
(1996)

FOREWORD by F.M.J. Debruyne	7
INTRODUCTION by J.J. Mattelaer	9
THE HISTORY OF UROLOGY IN FRANCE by A. Jardin	11
HIGHLIGHTS FROM THE HISTORY OF GREEK UROLOGY (from the late Bronze Age to the post-Byzantine period) by S.G. Marketos, A.A. Diamandopoulos, E. Poulakou-Rebelakou and C. Dimopoulos	35
THE HISTORY OF UROLOGY IN THE NETHERLANDS by J.D.M. De Vries	65
THE HISTORY OF UROLOGY IN CROATIA by D. Derezig	111
THE HISTORY OF UROLOGY IN FINLAND by K.J. Oravisto	119
THE HISTORY OF UROLOGY IN ROMANIA by E. Proca	127
AN INTRODUCTION TO METHODOLOGICAL PROBLEMS IN THE HISTORY OF UROLOGY by S. Musitelli, H. Jallous, C. Marandola and P. Marandola	137
OUTLINE OF A CRITICAL SURVEY OF UROLOGICAL HISTORIOGRAPHY by P. Marandola, S. Musitelli and H. Jallous	175
THE HISTORY OF BLADDER CATHETERISATION by J.J. Mattelaer	201

CONTENTS of VOLUME 4
de Historia Urologiae Europaeae
(1997)

FOREWORD by F.M.J. Debruyne	7
INTRODUCTION by J.J. Mattelaer	9
THE HISTORY OF UROLOGY IN THE EUROPEAN COUNTRIES	
THE HISTORY OF BULGARIAN UROLOGY by T. Patrashkov and C. Kumanov	15
THE HISTORY OF UROLOGY IN PORTUGAL by F. Calais Da Silva and A. Pinto De Carvalho	23
THE DEVELOPMENT OF UROLOGY IN DENMARK by V. Hvidt and L. Lauridsen	37
THE HISTORY OF UROLOGY IN NORWAY by B. Otnes	51
THE HISTORY OF UROLOGY IN SERBIA AND MONTENEGRO by J. Nikolic and D. Konjevic	65
THE HISTORY OF UROLOGY IN GREECE (from the post-Byzantine period to our days) by S.G. Marketos, E. Poulakou-Rebelakou, A. Rebelakos and C. Dimopoulos	87
THE HISTORY OF UROLOGY IN SWITZERLAND by D. Hauri	101
THE HISTORY OF THE E.O.R.T.C. by M. Pavone-Macaluso and P.H. Smith	119
HISTORICAL TALES OF UROLOGY	
UROLITHIASIS IN NON-MEDICAL BYZANTINE TEXTS by J. Lascaratos, E. Poulakou-Rebelakou and A. Rebelakos	155
THE EARLY (SURGICAL) HISTORY OF BLADDER CANCER by F. I. Chinegwundo	163
RESTORATION OF THE PREPUCE A HISTORICAL REVIEW by D. Schultheiss, M.C. Truss, C.G. Stief and U. Jonas	175
ERRATA: CORRECTIONS TO VOLUMES I, II and III by S. Musitelli	189

CONTENTS of VOLUME 5
de Historia Urologiae Europaeae
(1998)

FOREWORD by F.M.J. Debruyne	7
INTRODUCTION by J.J. Mattelaer	9
THE HISTORY OF UROLOGY IN THE EUROPEAN COUNTRIES	
THE MODERN HISTORY OF UROLOGY IN SPAIN SINCE THE RENAISSANCE by E. Maganto Pavon and R. Vela Navarrete	15
HIGHLIGHTS IN THE HISTORY OF UROLOGY IN GERMANY by P. Rathert, F. Moll and D. Schultheiss	45
THE HISTORY OF UROLOGY IN ALBANIA by F. Tartari	75
A BRIEF HISTORY OF UROLOGY IN SLOVAKIA by V. Zvara, J. Breza, M. Hor̃nák	97
THE HISTORY OF UROLOGY IN MALTA by P. Cassar	111
HISTORICAL TALES OF UROLOGY	
PHARMACOLOGICAL TREATMENT OF UROLOGICAL DISEASES IN THE ROMAN EMPIRE by S. Musitelli, H. Jallous, P. Marandola	131
THE HISTORY OF THE URODYNAMICS OF THE LOWER URINARY TRACT by J.J. Mattelaer	161
CIRCUMCISION: A SYMBOLIC ACT? A HISTORY AND ATTEMPTED INTERPRETATION by M. Libert	179
LITHOTOMY: ONE OF THE MOST MACABER CHAPTERS IN THE HISTORY OF UROLOGY by J. De Moerloose	209
TABLEAU DE L'OPERATION DE LA TAILLE BY MARIN MARAIS (1725) by S. Evers	235
UROLOGIC REFERENCES IN THE HOMERIC EPICS by E. Poulakou-Rebelakou, A.G. Rebelakos and S.G. Marketos	249
DE HISTORIA UROLOGIAE EUROPAEAE INDEX vol. 1-5 (1998) by Sergio Musitelli	

199

CONTENTS of VOLUME 6
de Historia Urologiae Europaeae
(1999)

FOREWORD by F.M.J. Debruyne   7

INTRODUCTION by J.J. Mattelaer   9

THE HISTORY OF UROLOGY IN THE EUROPEAN COUNTRIES

THE HISTORY OF UROSCOPY   19
(is in fact the history of medicine in Europe till the XVth century)
by J.J. Mattelaer

THE HISTORY OF UROLOGY IN GEORGIA   57
by L.G. Managadze, G.A. Gzirishvilli, T.I. Shioshvili, Z.M. Chanturaia

THE HISTORY OF UROLOGY IN TURKEY   69
by V. Solok, M. Çek

A BRIEF HISTORY OF UROLOGY IN LENINGRAD   89
by L.M. Gorilovski

THE DEVELOPMENT OF UROLOGY IN LITHUANIA   101
by K.K. Jocius, H. Ramonas, J. Mickevicius

THE HISTORY OF UROLITHIASIS AND ENDOSCOPY IN ALBANIA   121
by F. Tartari

HISTORICAL TALES OF UROLOGY

UROLOGY AND URINE IN BERNARDINO RAMAZZINI   133
by P. Marandola, S. Musitelli, H. Jallous

ANDROGEN THERAPY AND REJUVENATION IN THE EARLY 20TH CENTURY   141
by D. Schultheiss, J. Denil, U. Jonas

TRIBUTE TO ONE OF THE PIONEERS OF GREEK UROLOGICAL HISTORIOGRAPHY: 165
DR. SPYROS NAOUMIDIS (1907-1998)
by S.G. Marketos, E. Poulakou-Rebelakou, A. Rebelakos and C. Dimopoulos

LETTER TO THE EDITOR: 175
CONCERNING THE ARTICLE "RESTORATION OF
THE PREPUCE: A HISTORICAL REVIEW"
by F. Sorrentino, M. Sorrentino

CONTENTS of VOLUME 7
de Historia Urologiae Europaeae
(2000)

FOREWORD by F.M.J. Debruyne   7

INTRODUCTION by J.J. Mattelaer   9

THE HISTORY OF UROLOGY IN THE EUROPEAN COUNTRIES

THE HISTORY OF UROLOGY IN THE UKRAINE   15
by S.P. Pasechnikov

CURATIVE ATTEMPTS IN ILLNESSES OF THE URINARY ORGANS IN MEDIEVAL ICELAND 27
by C. Kaiser

FIFTY YEARS OF INTERSCANDINAVIAN UROLOGICAL COLLABORATION: 39
A RETROSPECTIVE VIEW
by Å. Fritjofson

HISTORICAL TALES OF UROLOGY

LITHOTOMY IN THE 18th AND 19th CENTURIES   51
by P.P. Figdor

ENDOSCOPIC LITHOTRIPSY OF URINARY BLADDER CALCULI   73
by M.A. Reuter

THE HISTORY OF TROCARS   85
by G. Seydl

LITHOTRIPSY IN AMERICA: TRANSFER OF THE TECHNIQUE FROM EUROPE (1824-1840) 95
by J.M. Edmonson

CHARLES V: AN INNOVATING UROLOGY PATIENT   109
by R. Vela Navarrete

HIGHLIGHTS IN THE HISTORY OF THE OPERATING MICROSCOPE   113
by J. Denil and D. Schultheiss

ROBERT PROUST - AN EMINENT DOCTOR IN THE   125
SHADOW OF HIS FAMOUS BROTHER MARCEL
by R. Speck

CONTENTS of VOLUME 8
de Historia Urologiae Europaeae
(2001)

FOREWORD by F.M.J. Debruyne — 7

INTRODUCTION by J.J. Mattelaer — 9

THE HISTORY OF UROLOGY IN THE EUROPEAN COUNTRIES

UROLOGY IN ESTONIA PAST AND PRESENT — 15
by Gennadi Timberg, Harry Tihane, Heiki Kask and
Eldor Mihkelsoo

THE HISTORY OF UROLOGY IN THE REPUBLIC — 31
OF MACEDONIA (FYROM)
by Stravidis Aleksander

EUROPE'S INFLUENCE ON AMERICAN UROLOGY — 39
IN THE 19th CENTURY
by Rainer M. Engel

HISTORICAL TALES OF UROLOGY

VIENNA: A TREASURY OF THE HISTORY OF MEDICINE AND UROLOGY — 61

by Johan J. Mattelaer

THE HISTORIC INTERACTION OF ANAESTHESIA — 73
AND UROLOGY
by Friedrich Moll, A. Karenberg and Peter Rathert

MALDESCENSUS TESTIS - THE HISTORY OF OPERATIVE TREATMENT — 95
by Knut Albrecht and Dirk Schultheiss

A REINVESTIGATION OF THE SIGNIFICANCE OF — 109
"BOMBOLZINI" IN THE HISTORY OF ENDOSCOPY
by Peter P. Figdor

THE HISTORY OF URINARY TRACT INFECTIONS — 119
by J. O. Elo

JOHN HUNTER: FOUNDER OF SCIENTIFIC UROLOGY AND PIONEER IN — 127
THE FIELD OF UROGENITAL SURGERY
by K. Skrepetis and N. Autoniou

OTTO KNEISE: A PIONEER OF MODERN — 137
UROLOGY
by Jürgen Konert

CONTENTS of VOLUME 9
de Historia Urologiae Europaeae
(2002)

FOREWORD by F.M.J. Debruyne — 7

INTRODUCTION by J.J. Mattelaer — 9

THE HISTORY OF UROLOGY IN THE EUROPEAN COUNTRIES

THE HISTORY OF UROLOGY IN BOHEMIA - PRAGUE — 15
by L. Jarolím

THE HISTORY OF UROLOGY IN SLOVENIA — 27
by Sedmak Boris and Trwinar Bojar

EUROPE'S INFLUENCE ON THE DEVELOPMENT OF SOUTH AMERICAN UROLOGY — 33
by E. Maganto Pavon

MODERN UROLOGISTS: WHERE DO YOU COME FROM? — 51
By P. Marandola, S. Musitelli and D.Vitetta.

HISTORICAL TALES OF UROLOGY FRANZ VON PAULA GRUITHUISEN (1774-1852) — 73
- HIS CONTRIBUTION TO THE DEVELOPMENT OF LITHOTRIPSY
by T. Zajaczkowski, A.M. Zamann and P. Rathert

FRANCESCO PAJOLA (1742-1816) - A PIONEER OF LITHOTOMY — 87
by P.P. Figdor

THE HISTORY OF RENAL ANATOMO-PHYSIOLOGY — 101
by S. Musitelli and J.J. Mattelaer

LEON KRYNSKI - EMINENT UROLOGIST OF THE LATE XIXth CENTURY — 131
- CREATOR OF SUBMUCOSAL TRANSPLANTATION OF THE URETERS INTO THE
SIGMOID COLON
by R. Sosnowski, T. Chwalinski, T. Demkow, A. Sródka

A 10th CENTURY MEDICAL DEONTOLOGIST, ISHAQ IBN ALI AL-RUHAWI, — 147
AND HIS STATEMENT ON BEVERAGES
by S. Aksoy and A.Verit

OPERATIVE UROLOGY AND THE HIPPOCRATIC OATH — 155
by P.F. Kalafatis, K.B. Zougdas, F.J. Dimitriadis and M.P. Kalafatis

COMMENT — 163
by S. Musitelli

LETTER TO THE EDITORS — 165

CONTENTS of VOLUME 10
de Historia Urologiae Europaeae
(2003)

FOREWORD by F.M.J. Debruyne   7

INTRODUCTION by J.J. Mattelaer   9

THE HISTORY OF UROLOGY IN THE EUROPEAN COUNTRIES

THE HISTORY OF UROLOGY IN THE REPUBLIC OF BELARUS   15
by A. Strotsky

UROLOGY IN THE MARIA HOSPITAL IN HELSINKI, FINLAND   25
by J. Elo and M. Ala-Opas

THE PEREGRINATIONS OF THE LICHTLEITER   35
by J.J. Mattelaer, M. Skopec, R. Engel and D. Schultheiss

WOMEN IN EUROPEAN UROLOGY   41
by M. Ruutu, J.J. Mattelaer and members of the EAU Historical Committee

HISTORICAL TALES OF UROLOGY

JULIUS BRUCK (1840-1902) - HIS CONTRIBUTION   59
TO THE DEVELOPMENT OF ENDOSCOPY
by T. Zajaczkowski, A.P. Zamann

UROLOGICAL TECHNIQUES OF SEREFEDDIN SABUNCUOGLU IN THE 15th CENTURY   83
OTTOMAN PERIOD
by A.Verit, S.Aksoy, H.Kafali and F.F.Verit

EVOLUTION OF VASOGRAPHY DURING 20th CENTURY   95
by K. Skrepetis, N. Antoniou

CASTRATION FROM MESOPOTAMIA TO THE XVIth CENTURY   111
by S. Musitelli and J.F. Felderhof

THE PROOF OF PATERNITY: THE HISTORY OF AN ANDROLOGICAL-FORENSIC   135
CHALLENGE
by K. Albrecht and D. Schultheiss

TABLE OF CONTENTS Volumes 1-9   147

CONTENTS of VOLUME 11
de Historia Urologiae Europaeae
(2004)

FOREWORD by F.M.J. Debruyne   7

INTRODUCTION by D. Schultheiss   9

THE HISTORY OF UROLOGY IN THE EUROPEAN COUNTRIES

THE 50th ANNIVERSARY OF THE FINNISH UROLOGICAL ASSOCIATION   13
by J. Elo and M. Ala-Opas

ETHICAL PRINCIPLES AND PRACTICE IN PEDIATRIC UROLOGICAL OPERATIONS IN   25
THE OTTOMAN EMPIRE
by S.N. Cenk Buyukunal and N. Sari

HISTORICAL TALES OF UROLOGY

HERMAPHRODISM AND ITS SURGICAL TREATMENT FROM ARISTOTLE   39
TO THE XV CENTURY
by S. Musitelli

SEMINAL STAINS IN LEGAL MEDICINE: A HISTORICAL REVIEW OF THE   51
FORENSICAL PROOF
by K. Albrecht and D. Schultheiss

THE UROGENITAL APPARATUS IN JUAN VALVERDE AND ANDREAS VESALIUS   65
by S. Musitelli

WILLIAM CHESELDEN, THE FATHER OF LITHOTOMY   81
by S. Wheatstone, B. Challacombe, P. Dasgupta

SIR HENRY THOMPSON: ARTIST, SCIENTIST, MOTORIST, GOURMET, TRAVELLER,   91
NOVELIST, CREMATIONIST AND SUB-SPECIALIST UROLOGIST
by J.C. Goddard and D.E. Osborn

NIKOLAJ A. BOGORAZ: RUSSIAN PIONEER OF PHALLOPLASTY AND PENILE   107
IMPLANT SURGERY
by A. Gabouev, U. Jonas, D. Schultheiss

GEZA ILLYÉS, FOUNDER OF HUNGARIAN UROLOGY   121
by I. Romics, Z. Fazakas, G. Nádas

ERRATA CORRIGE   133
by S. Musitelli

TABLE OF CONTENTS Volumes 1-10   135

CORRECTIONS TO VOLUME IX   152

205

CONTENTS of VOLUME 12
de Historia Urologiae Europaeae
(2005)

FOREWORD by P. Teilliac   9

INTRODUCTION by D. Schultheiss   11

THE HISTORY OF UROLOGY IN THE EUROPEAN COUNTRIES

THE HISTORY OF UROLOGY IN LATVIA   15
by I. Smiltens and E. Vjaters

THE DEVELOPMENT OF UROLOGY IN SZCZECIN: HOW POLITICAL CHANGES   23
INFLUENCED MEDICINE
by T. Zajaczkowski and E.M. Wojewski-Zajaczkowski

CZECHOSLOVAK-SWEDISH-FINNISH UROLOGICAL SYMPOSIA HELD BETWEEN   53
1969 AND 1988
by V. Zvara and J. Elo

ESTABLISHMENT AND DEVELOPMENT OF MODERN UROLOGY IN SYRIA: 61
FRENCH INFLUENCE AND SYRIAN INITIATIVE
by A. K. Chamssuddin

HISTORICAL TALES OF UROLOGY

A BRIEF SURVEY OF THE HISTORY OF SCIENTIFIC MUSEUMS FROM THE   73
15th TO THE 18th CENTURY
by S. Musitelli and H. Jallous

PALEOANDROLOGICAL ITEMS OF THE EARLIEST RELIGIOUS ARCHITECTURE: 91
9-10th MILLENNIUM BC
by A. Verit, C. Kurkcuoglu, F.F. Verit, H. Kafali and E. Yeni

THE FERTILITY GODDESS, CYBELE, AND ANDROLOGY   101
by C. Asvestis, A. Siatelis, D. Anagnostou, P. Karouzakis, E. Coralles and A. Tselikas

CHOCOLATE AND IMPOTENCE: AN HISTORICAL VIEW FROM EARLY SPANISH   113
DOCUMENTS AND BAROQUE LITERATURE
by R. Vela Navarrete

MALE GENITAL PATHOLOGY IN LEGAL MEDICINE: A HISTORICAL REVIEW   121
by K. Albrecht and D. Schultheiss

HISTORICAL REMARKS ON THE DIAGNOSIS AND TREATMENT OF HYDROCELES   143
by F.H. Moll and P. Rathert

THE LITHOSCOPE 153
by H-D. Nöske and E.W. Hauck

GEORG KELLING: THE MAN WHO INTRODUCED MODERN LAPAROSCOPY 163
INTO MEDICINE
by M. Hatzinger and J.K. Badawi

TERENCE MILLIN: A UROLOGICAL PIONEER 171
by D.M. Bouchier-Hayes

CONTENTS of VOLUME 13
de Historia Urologiae Europaeae
(2006)

FOREWORD by P. Teilliac	9
INTRODUCTION by D. Schultheiss	11
IN MEMORIAM: PROF. DR. LUDWIK JERZY MAZUREK by J. Mattelaer	13

THE HISTORY OF UROLOGY IN THE EUROPEAN COUNTRIES

THE HISTORY OF UROLOGY IN BOSNIA AND HERZEGOVINA by D. Aganovic	19

HISTORICAL TALES OF UROLOGY

A MAGNIFICENT CIRCUMCISION CARNIVAL IN THE EARLY 18th CENTURY OTTOMAN PERIOD by A. Verit, M. Cengiz, E. Yeni, D. Unal	37
KORO – THE PSYCHOLOGICAL DISAPPEARANCE OF THE PENIS by W. Jilek and J. Mattelaer	57
MASTURBATION AND MASS DELUSION: THE STORY OF SPERMATORRHOEA by D. Hodgson	75
THE LEGACY OF SPERMATORRHOEA A COMMENT ON THE ARTICLE BY D. HODGSON by F. Hodges	95
THE UROLOGICAL FATAL DISEASE OF THE BYZANTINE EMPEROR, JUSTIN II (565-578 AD) by E. Poulakou-Rebelakou, C. Alamanis, E. Koutsiaris, A. Rempelakos	101
HENRY DE TOULOUSE-LAUTREC AND JEAN ALFRED FOURNIER: A RELATIONSHIP ON CANVAS by L. Fariña	111
JOSEPH DIETL (1804-1878) HIS CONTRIBUTION TO THE ADVANCEMENT OF MEDICINE AND HIS CREDIT FOR UROLOGY by T. Zajaczkowski	125
A HISTORY OF CRYOSURGERY by S. Ahmed	145

CONTENTS of VOLUME 14
de Historia Urologiae Europaeae
(2007)

FOREWORD by P. Teillac 7

INTRODUCTION by D. Schultheiss 9

THE HISTORY OF UROLOGY IN EUROPEAN COUNTRIES

THE HISTORY OF UROLOGY IN ICELAND 13
by T. Gislason

HISTORICAL TALES OF UROLOGY

THE HISTORICAL JOURNEY OF THE PHALLUS FROM 10,000 BC 25
by M. Kendirci, Ö. Acar, U. Boylu, A. Kadioglu, C. Miroglu

THE URINARY TRACT IN GERMAN TEXTBOOKS OF LEGAL MEDICINE: 43
A HISTORICAL REVIEW OF 200 YEARS
by K. Albrecht, D. Schultheiss

UROLOGY AT NECKER HOSPITAL 1966: A SCANDINAVIAN VIEW 65
by J. Elo

MASTERS OF MICTURITION: THE FULLERS OF ANCIENT ROME 79
by J. R. Hill

HANS CHRISTIAN JACOBAEUS: THE INVENTOR OF HUMAN LAPAROSCOPY 95
AND THORACOSCOPY
by M. Hatzinger, S.T. Kwon, M. Sohn

THE MOMENT OF ENLIGHTENMENT 103
by R.C.M. Pelger

SIR PETER FREYER: A PIONEERING UROLOGIST 113
by J. P. O'Donoghue

THE ORIGINS OF SCIENTIFIC TREATMENT FOR VENEREAL DISEASES IN ATHENS IN THE 121
EARLY 20th CENTURY
by E. Poulakou-Rebelakou, C. Tsiamis, C. Alamanis, A. Rempelakos

JOHANN ANTON VON MIKULICZ-RADECKI 1850-1905): PROMOTER 135
(OF MODERN SURGERY AND CONTRIBUTION TO UROLOGY
by T. Zajaczkowski

THE HISTORY OF AN 85 YEAR OLD 165
EUROPEAN UROLOGICAL DEPARTMENT
by I. Romics, R. Engel, T. Stevens, P. Nyirády

CONTENTS of VOLUME 15
de Historia Urologiae Europaeae
(2008)

FOREWORD by P-A. Abrahamsson	7
INTRODUCTION by D. Schultheiss	9
THE HISTORY OF UROLOGY IN EUROPEAN COUNTRIES BERLIN'S INTERNATIONAL REPUTATION By Rainer Engel	11
PIONEERS IN UROLOGY By various authors	15
HISTORICAL TALES OF UROLOGY INFORMED CONSENT IN BLADDER STONE TREATMENT FROM THE OTTOMAN ARCHIVES By S. Aydın, A. Verit	27
CASTRATION: THE EUNUCHS OF QING DYNASTY CHINA: A MEDICAL AND HISTORICAL REVIEW By M. Bultitude, J. Chatterton	37
THE GREEK AND ROMAN PHALLIC INFLUENCE IN MEDIEVAL WESTERN EUROPE By J. J. Mattelaer	49
A BRIEF SURVEY OF THE HISTORY OF PEYRONIE'S DISEASE By S. Musitelli, M. Bossi, H. Jallous	73
WOLFGANG AMADEUS MOZART A UROLOGICAL PATHOGRAPHY By M. Hatzinger, S.T. Kwon	95
GENITOURINARY MEDICINE & SURGERY IN NELSON'S NAVY By J.C. Goddard	105
LUDWIG VON RYDYGIER: HIS CONTRIBUTION TO THE ADVANCEMENT OF SURGERY AND HIS CREDIT FOR UROLOGY By T. Zajaczkowski	123
STUDIES ON THE KIDNEY AND THE RENAL CIRCULATION, BY JOSEP TRUETA I RASPALL By L.A. Fariña	155
A MODERN POEM IN LATIN ON THE PROSTATE By J. J. Mattelaer	165
TABLE OF CONTENTS Volumes 1-14	169

CONTENTS of VOLUME 16
de Historia Urologiae Europaeae
(2009)

FOREWORD by P.-A. Abrahamsson   7

INTRODUCTION by D. Schultheiss   11

THE HISTORY OF UROLOGY IN EUROPEAN COUNTRIES

LEOPOLD CASPER, THE UROLOGICAL HERITAGE   15
By F. Moll and P. Rathert

COMBAT UROLOGY IN WORLD WAR II URINARY PATHOLOGY AT THE RUSSIAN   27
FRONT (191-1943)
By J.M. Poyato et al.

THE TUBERCULOSIS HOSPITAL IN HOHENKRUG, STETTIN DEPARTMENT OF   43
GENITOURINARY TUBERCULOSIS IN SZCZECIN-ZDUNOWO
By T. Zajaczkowski

IN THE SLIPSTREAM OF DR. KOLFF   67
By H. Broers

RESEARCH ON THE HISTORY OF EUROPEAN UROLOGY PAST, PRESENT AND FUTURE   83
By J. Elo, J. Mattelaer and D. Schultheiss

HISTORICAL TALES OF UROLOGY

CATHERINE DE MEDICI: THE CURE OF HER "INFERTILITY" AND SUBSEQUENT   105
CONTROL OF 16th CENTURY FRANCE
By J. Gordetsky and R. Rabinowitz

THE MANAGEMENT OF URETHRAL STRICTURES   119
IN ANCIENT INDIA THE ERA OF SUÇRUTA
By R. Nair et al.

HRÚTR HERJÓLFSSON: A VIKING TOO LARGE FOR HIS WIFE URO-OATHOLOGICAL   131
WORKUP OF A 1000 YEAR OLD STORY
By S. Buntrock and W. Heizmann

THE ETYMOLOGY OF CASTRATION AND ITS ASSOCIATION WITH   143
THE SELF-CASTRATING BEAVER
By A. R. Rao

THE MANAGEMENT OF PATIENTS WITH A URETHRAL ANOMALY A   155
DESCRIPTION IN A TEXTBOOK OF SURGERY PUBLISHED IN THE 18th CENTURY
By E.Yesildag and S.N.C. Buyukunal

WHEN THE PHALLUSSES WERE STILL GROWING ON TREES   167
By J.J. Mattelaer

CONTENTS of VOLUME 17
de Historia Urologiae Europaeae
(2010)

FOREWORD by P.-A. Abrahamsson　　　　　　　　　　　　　　　　　　　　7

INTRODUCTION by D. Schultheiss　　　　　　　　　　　　　　　　　　　　11

THE 4TH INTERNATIONAL CONGRESS ON THE HISTORY OF UROLOGY　　　15
By Reiner Engel

JAQUES-LOUIS REVERDIN (1842-1929): THE SURGEON AND THE NEEDLE　　25
By Luis A. Fariña-Pérez

A HISTORICAL REVIEW OF FOURNIER'S GANGRENE　　　　　　　　　　　37
By José Medina Polo, Ana González-Rivas Fernández and Óscar Leíva Galvis

JOHN HUNTER'S UROLOGIC DRAWINGS　　　　　　　　　　　　　　　　51
By Michael E. Moran

PATTISON FASCIA: THE FORGOTTEN EPONYM?　　　　　　　　　　　　　63
By Dirk Schultheiss

DO UNTO YOURSELF AS YOU WOULD DO TO OTHERS –
SELF EXPERIMENTATION IN UROLOGY　　　　　　　　　　　　　　　　77
By Johanna Thomas, Omer Karim, Hanif Motiwala and Amrith Raj Rao

HISTORY OF THE TERM PROSTATE　　　　　　　　　　　　　　　　　　91
Franz Josef Marx and Axel Karenberg

ANDREAS VESALIUS AND SEMINAL ERRORS　　　　　　　　　　　　　　105
By Michael E. Moran

THE LEGEND OF SUN SHIMIAO: THE MAN WHO INVENTED URETHRAL
CATHETERIZATION　　　　　　　　　　　　　　　　　　　　　　　　　119
By Wei Wang and Peter M. Thompson

A SHORT HISTORY OF "ORIENTAL TESTIS"　　　　　　　　　　　　　　129
By S.N. Cenk Buyukunal and Ayten Altıntaş

THE RELATIONSHIP BETWEEN THE PHYSICIAN　　　　　　　　　　　　　141
AND THE INSTRUMENT MAKER
By Michaela Zykan

TABLES OF CONTENTS　　　　　　　　　　　　　　　　　　　　　　　　151
Volumes 1-16

CONTENTS of VOLUME 18
de Historia Urologiae Europaeae
(2011)

Foreword by Per-Anders Abrahamsson	9
Introduction by Dirk Schultheiss	12
THE HISTORY OF UROLOGY IN EUROPEAN COUNTRIES	
RECORDING HISTORY- THE LIVING WITNESS PROGRAMME By Dominic Hodgson and Peter Thompson	15
THE SECOND OLDEST UROLOGICAL DEPARTMENT IN EUROPE IS 90 YEARS OLD By Attila Szendröi, Imre Romics	29
EDUCATION IN MEDICINE AND SURGERY - DEVELOPMENT OF UROLOGY IN DANZIG/GDAN'SK By Thaddaeus Zajaczkowski	49
HISTORICAL TALES OF UROLOGY	
CIRCUMCISION AND GENITAL DECORATION AS FIRST UROLOGICAL INTERVENTIONS DURING PALEOLITHIC TIMES By Javier Angulo and Marcos García-Díez	81
AMPULLAE DUCTUS DEFERENTIS, SEMINAL VESICLES AND PROSTATE GLAND IN THE HELLENISTIC ANATOMISTS AND GALEN By Sergio Musitelli and Ilaria Bossi, with comments by Franz J. Marx and Axel Karenberg	97
LITHOTOMISTS AND THEIR EX LIBRIS By Dirk Mattelaer	119
PALEOLITHOLOGY By Michael E. Moran	129
DE URINIS TRACTATUS DUO BY H.J. REGA By Johan Mattelaer	139
THE HISTORY OF PERCUTANEOUS NEPHROLITHOTOMY - THROUGH THE KEYHOLE TO A WIDER WORLD By Alistair Rogers, Toby Page and Peter English	153
CIRCUMCISION AND SUBINCISION IN AUSTRALIAN ABORIGINAL TRIBES By Rachel Thomson and Matthew Bultitude	165
LITHOTOMISTS AT THE DAWN OF THE UNITED STATES By Rainer Engel	173
UROPOIESIS: GALEN AGAINST ERASÍSTRATUS AND ASCLEPÍADES By Sergio Musitelli and Ilaria Bossi	189
ALEXANDER VON LICHTENBERG (1880-1949): SCHOLAR, PHYSICIAN, MIGRANT By Matthis Krischel amd Friedrich Moll	203
SLAVES TO AN EMPRESS: J. MARION SIMS, VESICO-VAGINAL FISTULA REPAIR, AND SURGICAL EXPERIMENTATION By Sara Spettel and Sakti Das	215
TABLES OF CONTENTS Volumes 1-17	229

CONTENTS of VOLUME 19
de Historia Urologiae Europaeae
(2012)

FOREWORD by P.-A. Abrahamsson   7

FOREWORD by Per-Anders Abrahamsson   9

INTRODUCTION by Dirk Schultheiss   12

THE HISTORY OF UROLOGY IN EUROPEAN COUNTRIES

JEWISH UROLOGISTS UNDER NATIONAL SOCIALISM – A CALL TO SUPPORT   15
A NEW EAU RESEARCH PROJECT !
Dirk Schultheiss

THE INFLUENCE OF HUNGARIAN-BORN PHYSICIANS ON THE DEVELOPMENT OF   19
MEDICINE IN VIENNA
Manfred Skopec

UROLOGY IN LWÓW, LEMBERG AND LVIV: HOW POLITICAL CHANGES INFLUENCED   35
THE DEVELOPMENT OF MEDICINE AND UROLOGY. STANISŁAW LASKOWNICKI
(1892-1978)-THE FIRST PROFESSOR OF UROLOGY IN POLAND
Thaddaeus Zajaczkowski

HISTORICAL TALES IN UROLOGY

VARICOCELE IN ANCIENT GREEK ART AND SOCIETY   73
Sergio Musitelli, Ilaria Bossi

MEN WITH BREASTS! HISTORY OF GYNAECOMASTIA THROUGHOUT THE CENTURIES   83
Johan J. Mattelaer

ECHOES OF GREEK MYTHOLOGY IN UROLOGICAL TERMINOLOGY AND PRACTICE   115
E. Poulakou-Rebelakou, C. Tsiamis, C. Alamanis, A. Rempelakos

ON GIROLAMO FRACASTORO'S ALLEGED FOUNDATION OF MODERN "EPIDEMIOLOGY"   125
Sergio Musitelli, Ilaria Bossi

THE EMINENT VENEREOLOGIST PHILIPPE RICORD (1800-1899) AND HIS   137
LANDMARK WORK ON SYPHILIS
M. Karamanou, E. Poulakou-Rebelakou, L. Rempelakos, A. Rempelakos, G. Androutsos

AUGUSTE NÉLATON (1807-1873): AN IMPORTANT UROLOGIST "AVANT LA LETTRE"   145
Philip E.V. Van Kerrebroeck

TRAITÉ DES MALADIES DES VOIES URINAIRES   169
BY PIERRE DESAULT AND XAVIER BICHAT PUBLISHED IN 1799 A REPRESENTATIVE
DISCOURSE OF THE PROTOUROLOGY PERIOD
Norberto M. Fredotovich

SIR PERCIVALL POTT AND HIS MEMORABLE CONTRIBUTION TO THE 187
EPIDEMIOLOGY OF THE CHIMNEY SWEEPER'S CANCER
V. Hanchanale, A.R. Rao

VICTOR IVÁNCHICH: PIONEER OF ACADEMIC UROLOGY 203
Manfred Skopec and Michael Marberger

CENTENARY OF JOSEPH BELL (1837-1911): THE SURGEON WHO INSPIRED 213
SHERLOCK HOLMES
Luis A. Fariña-Pérez

KIRILL SAPEZHKO: THE 19TH CENTURY PIONEER IN ORAL MUCOSA GRAFTS 225
TRANSPLANTATION
Igor Korneyev, Dmitry Ilyin, Dirk Schultheiss

ALBERT HOGGE (1867-1933), THE FIRST PROFESSOR OF UROLOGY IN BELGIUM 239
Jean de Leval

THE GRAND CHARLATAN 247
Rainer M. Engel

PROFESSOR SIR LUDWIG GUTTMANN (1899-1980): A NEW APPROACH TO SPINAL 267
INJURED PATIENTS
John Henderson

WHO OPENED PANDORA'S BOX? A HISTORICAL EVALUATION OF THE DIAGNOSIS 275
OF PROSTATE CANCER OVER THE COURSE OF A CENTURY
Caroline M Moore, Mark Emberton

HAROLD HOPKINS AND KARL STORZ – THE PHYSICIST AND AN INSTRUMENT 285
MAKER
Jaimin Bhatt, Neil Haldar, Adam Jones, Sunil Kumar

TABLES OF CONTENTS VOLUMES 1-18 299

2013
ISBN/EAN: 978-90-815102-4-0
Printed by Drukkerij Gelderland
Arnhem, the Netherlands
© History Office EAU

For extra copies of this series:
History Office EAU
P.O. Box 30016
6803 AA Arnhem
The Netherlands

Front cover:
Ape with a urine flask. Stained glass window, York Minster.

Text correction:
Loek Keizer

No part of this publication may be reproduced, stored in a retrieval system, or transmitted by any means, electronic, mechanical or photocopying without written permission from the copyright holder.